THE CRA

THE CRANIAL NERVES

NERVES

Anatomy and anatomico-clinical correlations

by

ALF BRODAL
M.D.

Professor of Anatomy
University of Oslo, Norway

Translated from the Norwegian
by the author

SECOND EDITION

SIXTH PRINTING

BLACKWELL SCIENTIFIC PUBLICATIONS
OXFORD LONDON EDINBURGH MELBOURNE

Original title: *Hjernenervene*. Publ. in the series: 'Bibliotheca Medica'
by Ejnar Munksgaard, Copenhagen — C. W. K. Gleerup, Lund —
Johan Grundt Tanum, Oslo.

ISBN 0 632 00590 4

First Printed 1959
Reprinted 1962
Second Edition 1965
Reprinted 1967, 1969, 1972, 1976, 1978

Printed and bound in Great Britain
at the Alden Press, Oxford

Foreword to the Original Edition

AT first sight, it may seem hazardous to undertake the preparation of a monograph on the cranial nerves. The subject is a restricted one, even within the field of neurology, and the question arises as to whom such a book should be primarily addressed: the student, the general practitioner, the non-neurological specialist, or those who are daily concerned with organic disease of the nervous system? Will not many items necessarily be dealt with in too detailed a manner for one group of readers, while the same information will be superfluous for others?

This book settles any doubts on these questions. It may not be necessary for the candidate for medical examinations to know everything which the book contains, while the neurologist is — or ought to be — well acquainted with the fundamentals of the subject. Yet, for all the groups mentioned, this monograph represents a welcome addition to the Scandinavian medical literature, not only because it contains all relevant knowledge in this field necessary for each, but because it also integrates the anatomical, functional and clinical aspects of the subject.

These features of Professor Alf Brodal's treatment of the cranial nerves are characteristic of the wide range of his knowledge and interests. While at the same time pursuing original anatomo-physiological research, he manages to give short yet comprehensive descriptions of the structure, functions, and disfunctions of the nervous system, and this of a quality which is not common either on the Scandinavian or the international level. His *Nevro-anatomi i relasjon til klinisk nevrologi* of 1943, and the revised English version of 1948 (*Neurological Anatomy in Relation to Clinical Medicine*), are

5

standard works from which every student and doctor may profit, and to which every neurologist may turn with confidence for information.

It is to be hoped that this book will be the first of a series of similar works, both in neurology and in other fields of medicine; and that these monographs may help to re-create that integrated insight into medicine as a whole, which is in so much danger of being lost in the ever-increasing fragmentation of the subject into narrow specialities.

Mogens Fog, M.D.
Professor of Neurology,
University of Copenhagen

Preface to the First Edition

THE English edition of this book has been translated from the Norwegian, and in general follows this very closely. Some data from research done since 1956 have been included. The labellings of some of the illustrations have had to be translated, otherwise the illustrations have not been altered.

I am indebted to Dr David Bowsher, Department of Anatomy, University of Liverpool, for going through my translation and for correcting some errors and suggesting improvements in the wording.

Oslo, November 1958

A. BRODAL

Preface to the Second Edition

SOME recent data on the anatomy and physiology of the cranial nerves, particularly the stato-acoustic, have been included in the new edition. Figure 10 has been slightly altered in accordance with new findings. Otherwise the text and illustrations are as in the first edition.

Oslo, September 1964

A. BRODAL

Preface to the Original Edition

BIBLIOTHECA MEDICA has felt that in the Nordic countries there is a need for a description of the cranial nerves for the use of students and physicians. The aim of the present book, therefore, is to give a brief account of the anatomy of the cranial nerves, with particular emphasis on items of practical interest for clinical medicine. Since the cranial nerves and their functions cannot be understood except when evaluated in relation to the central nervous system as a whole, some features of the central connexions of the cranial nerves are included. The common symptoms occurring in diseases affecting the cranial nerves and their central connexions are briefly dealt with.

No attempt is made in this book to give an exhaustive presentation of all symptoms and variations of symptom constellations which may occur in diseases of the cranial nerves. Their anatomy explains why these variations are almost innumerable. A description which covers all of them, would, therefore, by far exceed the limits set for books in this series. However, knowing the anatomy and function of the various cranial nerves, the physician will be able logically to deduce the seat of damage to them. In the author's opinion this is a sounder and more reliable procedure than to attempt to make a given series of symptoms fit into one of the many syndromes which have been described (and which only rarely occur in their typical form). For this reason emphasis is put on the description of the anatomical and functional features. These will have to form the basis for any clinical reasoning in a particular case. Some special symptom-complexes which are seen fairly frequently are treated in an appendix.

References to original works are given to some extent, and

these chiefly to results of recent research. References to older works will be found in those listed.

For technical reasons it is only possible to bring a restricted number of simple diagrams to illustrate important anatomical data. For more complete illustrations the reader is referred to anatomical atlases. Some of the illustrations have been specially made for this book. Others have been borrowed from papers of other authors or from my own previous publications.

For the preparation of the illustrations I am indebted to the artist of the Anatomical Institute, Miss S. Mörch. My thanks are due to Miss O. Gorset for typing and secretarial assistance and to Dr Kr. Kristiansen, Oslo City Hospital, for going through the manuscript and for kind advice concerning the clinical features which are discussed in the text.

Oslo, May 1956

A. BRODAL

Contents

The Cranial Nerves in General

The name *cranial* or *cerebral nerves* is used for those peripheral nerves which leave the brain stem, to distinguish them from the spinal nerves which take their origin from the spinal cord and supply the neck, trunk and extremities. From ancient times it is customary to subdivide the cranial nerves into 12 pairs and to number them as follows: 1. The olfactory nerve. 2. The optic nerve. 3. The oculomotor nerve. 4. The trochlear nerve. 5. The trigeminal nerve. 6. The abducent nerve. 7. The facial nerve with the intermediate nerve. 8. The stato-acoustic nerve (representing the vestibular and cochlear nerves). 9. The glossopharyngeal nerve. 10. The vagus nerve. 11. The accessory nerve. 12. The hypoglossal nerve. For didactic reasons they will be considered in the reverse order in this book.

On account of the high degree of differentiation in the anterior part of the organism, not least on account of the development of the special sense organs in the head, the cranial nerves are more complex with regard to their structure and function than the spinal nerves. However, the two first pairs, the olfactory and optic nerves, are not cranial nerves in the proper sense. The optic nerve, for example, is actually to be compared to a tract within the central nervous system, which during development has been 'drawn out' from it. For practical reasons, these two nerves will be included in the following account. But they have to be left out of consideration when in this chapter some general features in the organization of the cranial nerves are to be dealt with. A knowledge of such general features will facilitate the comprehension of the individual cranial nerves.

In spite of certain differences between the cranial nerves proper, there are common features in their organization. When all the cranial nerves are considered together it turns out that they are made up of the same functional types of fibres as the spinal nerves. Before considering the cranial nerves, it will, therefore, be appropriate to recall the somewhat simpler situation in the spinal cord.

As will be known, each spinal nerve is formed by the fusion of a ventral (anterior) and a dorsal (posterior) root (fig. 1). The fibres making up the ventral roots emerge as a series of filaments laterally on the ventral surface of the spinal cord, while those forming the dorsal roots emerge laterally on its dorsal surface. The fibre bundles which fuse to form one spinal nerve are derived from a disc-shaped part of the cord referred to as a spinal segment.

The *ventral roots* consist exclusively of fibres which conduct impulses in a centrifugal direction, that is from the cord to the periphery. These fibres have their perikarya (cell bodies, somata) in the grey matter of the cord and are called *efferent*. All fibres in the *dorsal roots* conduct impulses in a centripetal direction, that is from the periphery to the cord. They are thus *afferent*, and have their perikarya in the spinal ganglia which appear as swellings on the dorsal roots. These perikarya are pseudo-unipolar nerve cells, and emit a single axon which dichotomizes in a T-shaped manner, one branch coursing to the periphery and the other passing into the cord (fig. 1). The latter branch synapses with other nerve cells in the grey matter of the spinal cord (or with the cells in the nuclei of the dorsal columns).

Within the two groups of fibres, efferent and afferent, a further subdivision can be made according to the type of structures which they supply peripherally. Fibres which innervate skeletal muscles, tendons, joints and ligaments are called *somatic*. To this group belong also most of the sensory fibres from the skin. *Visceral* fibres are those which innervate internal organs, smooth muscles, vessels and glands. Since both groups of organs may receive impulses from the cord as well as send impulses to it, there will be altogether 4 fibre categories: *somatic afferent*, *somatic efferent*, *visceral afferent* and *visceral efferent*.

Most of the *somatic efferent fibres in the spinal nerves* are relatively thick (broken lines in fig. 1). The majority are axons from the ventral motor horn cells, large multipolar nerve cells with coarse Nissl granules. The fibres leave the spinal cord in the ventral roots and course in the branches of those nerves

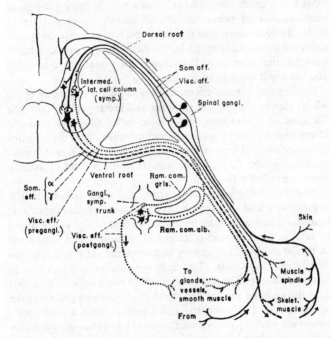

Fig. 1. Diagram of the fibre components of the spinal nerves. Description in text.

which supply skeletal muscle. Finally each nerve fibre splits into numerous fine branches, each of which ends in a motor end-plate on a single muscle fibre. It follows from this that a single motor ventral horn cell innervates a number of muscle fibres, actually 30-300 or more. If a particular ventral horn cell discharges it will cause all the muscle fibres which it supplies to contract. A motor ventral horn cell, its axon and all muscle fibres which it supplies constitute what Sherrington called a *motor unit*. This is the smallest functional unit in the motor apparatus. It is obvious that a muscle which is made up of many small units will be capable of performing smaller and more finely graded movements than a muscle having the same total number of fibres distributed among fewer but larger units. In agreement with this it has been found that the motor units are particularly small in, for example, the mimetic facial muscles, the muscles of the larynx, the external eye muscles and the small muscles of the hand.

Among the somatic efferent fibres there are some thin ones, which supply the muscle spindles and are capable of altering the state of contraction of their (so-called intrafusal) muscle fibres, and in this way to change the susceptibility of the spindles to stretching. These fibres are commonly referred to as γ-fibres, while the coarser ones to the (extrafusal) muscle fibres are called α-fibres.

The *visceral efferent fibres* from the cord belong to the sympathetic and parasympathetic divisions of the autonomic system. The *sympathetic fibres* (dotted line in fig. 1) are axons of cells in the intermediolateral cell column which is situated in the lateral horn of the grey matter in the 1st thoracic to the 2nd lumbar segments. The cells are smaller and less rich in Nissl substance than the ventral motor horn cells. The axons pass through the ventral horn to the ventral roots and enter the spinal nerve. From this the axons pass through a white communicant ramus (ramus communicans albus) to the sympathetic trunk, where they terminate in one of its ganglia. The impulses are here transmitted to multipolar nerve cells which send their axons either via a grey communicant ramus (ramus communicans griseus) back to a spinal nerve, in which they run to the periphery. Or the axons follow larger arteries in the peripheral direction. The latter fibres supply vessels and internal organs, the former pass to vessels, sweat glands and the smooth muscles attached to hairs in the skin. The *parasympathetic visceral efferent fibres* from the spinal cord are derived from the 2nd-4th sacral segments. They course peripherally in the corresponding spinal nerves to end in autonomic, visceral ganglia or plexuses which are found within or in the vicinity of the organs which they supply (for example the urinary bladder and the rectum). The cells of these ganglia, like those in the ganglia of the sympathetic trunk, are multipolar and have numerous long dendrites and an axon which runs to the organ to be innervated.

It will be seen from this that the *visceral efferent pathway from the cord to the various organs is made up of two successive neurons*. This applies to the sympathetic as well as to the parasympathetic system. The first link in the chain, the fibres from the cord to an autonomic ganglion, are called *preganglionic*; the second link, the fibres from the ganglion to the organ, are referred to as *postganglionic*.[1]

There are thus clear anatomical and functional distinctions between the somatic and visceral efferent fibres. With regard to the afferent fibres the distinction is less marked. The *somatic afferent* fibres (heavy line in fig. 1) come from such structures as the various types of sensory end organs in the skin, from nerve plexuses around the hairs, from Vater-Pacinian corpuscles, muscle spindles and tendon organs. Many of these fibres are relatively thick. They have their perikarya in the spinal ganglia. The central process of their perikarya may establish synaptical contact with cells in the dorsal horn of the spinal cord, and the axons of the latter cells may then transmit the sensory impulses to higher levels. Or the central process of the cells in the spinal ganglia may ascend in the dorsal funiculus and end around second order sensory neurons in the nuclei of the dorsal funiculi (nucleus gracilis and cuneatus). In addition to providing pathways for the

[1] At the termination of all preganglionic fibres and of the para-sympathetic postganglionic fibres liberation of acetylcholine takes place on passage of the impulses. At the termination of the sympathetic postganglionic fibres sympathin (closely related to adrenaline) is liberated (an exception being, however, the fibres to the sweat glands). The terms *cholinergic* and *adrenergic* fibres are, therefore, sometimes used for the two types.

conduction of sensory impulses to higher levels of the central nervous system, the somatic afferent fibres take part in the formation of reflex arcs (see fig. 1) by sending branches to cells in the grey matter of the cord. These cells send their axon in a ventral direction and synapse with ventral motor horn cells or other kinds of effector neurons. Some somatic afferent fibres pass directly to the ventral motor horn cells and take part in the arc of the tendon (myotatic) reflexes, which thus is a two-neuron (monosynaptic) reflex arc.

The *visceral afferent fibres* (thin line in fig. 1) are derived from visceral organs and vessels. No distinction can be made between sympathetic and parasympathetic afferent fibres. Whether in their central course they follow the sympathetic or parasympathetic efferent fibres, the visceral afferent ones all have their perikarya in the spinal ganglia. The central process of their cells enters the grey matter of the cord, and their further connexions, as far as is known, correspond largely to those of the somatic afferent fibres.

Turning now to the *cranial nerves*, we find the same principles in their organization as in the spinal nerves. There are thus in the cranial nerves *somatic afferent fibres* which transmit impulses from the skin and mucous membranes in the head to the brain stem. Just as the somatic afferent fibres in the spinal nerves have their perikarya in ganglia outside the central nervous system, the somatic afferent fibres in the cranial nerves have similar extracerebral ganglia. The cells in these ganglia are bipolar or pseudo-unipolar, and give off one branch to the brain stem, another to the periphery. The largest of these somatic afferent ganglia is the semilunar ganglion, belonging to the trigeminal nerve.

The fibres which have been described here are frequently called *general* somatic afferent, to distinguish them from fibres transmitting impulses from the special sense organs, the receptor organs in the inner ear. These are called *special* somatic afferent. (The fibres of the optic nerve are also special somatic afferent.) This type of fibre is not found in the spinal nerves.

The *visceral afferent fibres* in the cranial nerves conduct

18

afferent messages from internal organs such as the heart, lungs and stomach. These fibres also have their perikarya in ganglia, but while the visceral afferent fibres in the spinal nerves have their perikarya in the spinal ganglia, those of the cranial nerves have ganglia separate from those of the somatic afferent fibres. The largest of these ganglia is the nodose ganglion which belongs to the vagus nerve.

Like the somatic afferent fibres, the visceral afferent fibres may be subdivided into *general* visceral afferent from internal organs in general, and *special* visceral afferent fibres from visceral sense organs, namely the organs of taste. (The olfactory fibres are also special visceral afferent.)

The efferent fibres in the cranial nerves, like those of the spinal nerves, are of two types, visceral and somatic. The *visceral efferent fibres* take origin in nerve cells which are aggregated to form particular nuclei, just as do the visceral efferent fibres in the spinal nerves. The nerve cells in these nuclei are of the same type as those in the intermediolateral cell column in the cord, being medium sized and multipolar. The largest of the visceral efferent cranial nerve nuclei is the dorsal motor (parasympathetic) nucleus of the vagus. All visceral efferent fibres in the cranial nerves belong to the parasympathetic system. Just like the corresponding fibres from the cord, they do not pass directly to those organs which they innervate, but terminate in groups or collections of more scattered nerve cells which form *autonomic (visceral) ganglia*. The axons of these cells then run as postganglionic fibres to the various organs.

The *somatic efferent fibres* in the cranial nerves correspond to those fibres in the spinal nerves which are derived from the motor ventral horn cells and pass to skeletal musculature. The nuclei from which these fibres are derived are composed of large, multipolar nerve cells, with abundant and coarse Nissl granules.

Within this type of neurone a subdivision can be made according to whether the musculature to be innervated is developed from the mesenchyme of the visceral, branchial, arches or from myotomes of

19

the head. Strictly speaking, only the latter group of fibres corresponds to the somatic efferent fibres of the spinal nerves. They, like their nuclei of origin are, therefore, sometimes spoken of as *general* somatic efferent. To this group belongs, for example, the nucleus of the hypoglossal nerve. *Special* somatic efferent are the nuclei and fibres which supply muscles derived from the branchial arches, such as the motor nuclei and efferent fibres of the facial and trigeminal nerves.[1]

In table I the fibre components of the cranial nerves are listed. The table shows in which nerves the various types of fibre are present.

It will be seen from the table that there are wide variations between the cranial nerves with regard to the types of fibres which they carry. In agreement with this, in many of them it is not possible, as in the spinal nerves, to distinguish a motor and sensory root. The vagus nerve contains fibres of all types, afferent and efferent, somatic and visceral, while on the other hand the hypoglossal nerve and the abducent and trochlear nerves have only somatic efferent fibres, and the stato-acoustic nerve is purely somatic sensory. To some extent these differences are a secondary feature, due to the reduction of some components of some nerves during foetal development. On the other hand a definite order can be recognized in the topographical arrangement of the various cranial nerve nuclei. Those nuclei which are related to a particular type of fibre are arranged as a longitudinal column. It will be seen from figs. 2 and 3 that the *nuclei supplying the muscles of myotomic origin* (the nuclei of the hypoglossal, abducent, trochlear and oculomotor nerves) are situated close to the midline, just beneath the floor of the 4th ventricle and the aqueduct. Lateral to this column is another, consisting of the *nuclei which innervate the branchial musculature*, the special somatic efferent nuclei of the trigeminal, facial and vagus nerves (nucleus ambiguus). During foetal development, however, these nuclei have migrated in a ventral direction, but they have retained their longitudinal orientation. Then follows laterally the column of *visceral efferent nuclei*. This consists of the

[1] Some authors prefer to call this group of fibres special *visceral* efferent (see Herrick, 1943).

Table I

The fibre components of the cranial nerves

Afferent	1. Somatic	a. general, from skin and mucous membranes	N. V, VII, IX, X
		b. special, from the sensory organs in the inner ear	N. VIII
	2. Visceral	a. general, from internal organs	N. VII, IX, X
		b. special, from the organs of taste	N. VII, IX, X
Efferent	3. Visceral	to glands, vessels and smooth muscles	N. III, VII, IX, X
	4. Somatic	a. general, to muscles derived from the myotomes	N. III, IV, VI, XII
		b. special, to muscles derived from the branchial arches	N. V, VII, IX, X, (?)XI

dorsal motor nucleus of the vagus, the small inferior (medullary) and superior (pontine) salivatory nuclei, belonging to the glossopharyngeal and intermediate nerves, respectively, and finally the Edinger-Westphal nucleus of the oculomotor nerve. These nuclei are also situated just beneath the floor of the ventricular system. In the floor of the 4th ventricle, the *sulcus*

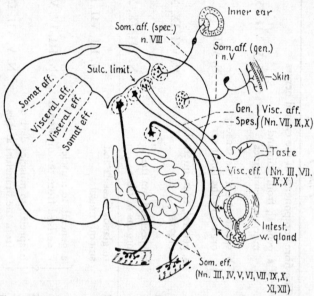

Fig. 2. The nuclei of origin and termination of the various types of fibres in the cranial nerves, as seen in a diagram of a cross-section through the medulla oblongata. (Redrawn from Strong and Elwyn.)

limitans (fig. 2) marks the border between a medial area, containing all the efferent nuclei, and a lateral area, where the terminal nuclei of all afferent, sensory, cranial nerve fibres are situated. Most medially in the sensory area is the large *visceral afferent nucleus*, the nucleus of the solitary tract, then follow the general somatic afferent nuclei: the three subdivisions of the sensory trigeminal nucleus. Most laterally, in

22

the floor of the lateral recess of the 4th ventricle, are the *special somatic afferent nuclei* of the cochlear and vestibular nerves.

Unlike the nuclei of origin of the efferent fibres, the terminal nuclei of the visceral and somatic afferent fibres form continuous columns. This has been explained by assuming that fibres

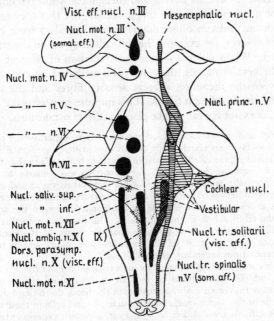

Fig. 3. Diagram showing the position of the various groups of cranial nerve nuclei in the brain stem. (From Brodal, 1949.)

transmitting the same type of impulses have a tendency to join each other and to terminate in the same region.

The nuclei of origin and termination of the cranial nerves are in the first place stations in the pathways for impulses from higher levels of the central nervous system to the effector organs and in the centrally directed pathways from the periphery to higher levels. Descending fibres from higher

23

parts of the central nervous system, first and foremost fibres of the 'pyramidal tract', mediate effects on the nuclei of origin.[1] From the sensory cranial nerve nuclei secondary fibres transmit sensory messages in a rostral direction within the brain stem. It is, however, important to be aware of the fact that the cranial nerves and their nuclei subserve not only conscious, sensory and motor, processes, but that they are also important links in numerous reflexes. Impulses from higher reflex centres, for example the colliculi, may act on the effector nuclei. When reflexes occur on stimulation of afferent fibres in the cranial nerves, these must be mediated by connexions between the incoming afferent sensory fibres and the nuclei giving rise to efferent fibres. This impulse transmission, however, does not appear to take place via direct connexions.

Neither in normal anatomical material nor in experimental studies has it so far been conclusively shown that primary sensory fibres of the cranial nerves establish synaptical contact with cells in the efferent nuclei. Szentágothai (1948a), for example, was unable to trace experimentally transected fibres of the trigeminal, vagus and glosso-pharyngeal nerves in the cat to any of the motor cranial nerve nuclei. Thus at least one neuron must be intercalated between the afferent and the efferent link in the reflex arcs. Our knowledge on this point is still incomplete. It is possible that the intercalated neurons in question may be cells of the reticular formation, which receive collaterals from secondary sensory fibres.

In a corresponding manner, the descending fibres in the pyramidal tract, which are assumed to mediate the impulses giving rise to voluntary movements of the muscles in the head, do not end directly on cells in the motor cranial nerve nuclei, but on cells in their neigh-bourhood. At least this is so in the cat, as shown experimentally by Walberg (1957b) and Szentágothai and Rajkovits (1958). This is analogous to the arrangement in the spinal cord, where at least 80 per cent of the fibres of the pyramidal tract end on intercalated neurons, and only very few synapse directly with ventral motor horn cells.

[1] It may be appropriate to emphasize that the 'pyramidal tract' according to recent studies is far more than the sum of efferent fibres from the giant cells of Betz in the precentral motor cortex. According to Lassek (1940, 1942) these account for some 2-3 per cent only of all fibres of the tract, which receives fibres from extensive parts of the cerebral cortex (for a recent discussion see for example Brodal, 1953; Walberg and Brodal, 1953).

24

Not only the motor, but also the sensory cranial nerve nuclei, are, however, under control of higher levels of the nervous system. Just as impulses from the cerebral cortex are able to inhibit the central propagation of sensory impulses entering the cord in the spinal nerves by acting on the first synaptic relay in the dorsal horns (Hagbarth and Kerr, 1954) by way of presynaptic inhibition (Andersen, Eccles and Sears, 1962), sensory impulses entering via the trigeminal nerve may be depressed in the same way (Hernández-Peón and Hagbarth, 1955). The anatomical basis for effects of this kind presumably are fibres from the cerebral cortex which have recently been shown experimentally to enter into synaptical contact with cells of the sensory trigeminal nuclei and the nucleus of the solitary tract (Brodal, Szabo and Torvik, 1956). In a similar way corticofugal fibres end also in the nuclei of the dorsal columns (Walberg, 1957a; Kuypers, 1958).

The nuclei of the cranial nerves are more or less surrounded by the *reticular formation of the brain stem* and have intimate functional relations with this. Thus secondary fibres from the sensory cranial nerve nuclei give off collaterals to cells in the reticular formation.

Such collaterals appear to mediate impulses to the so-called *ascending reticular activating system* of Moruzzi and Magoun (1949). This 'system' has been shown to transmit impulses via certain cell groups of the thalamus to extensive parts of the cerebral cortex, and to be essential for the maintenance of consciousness (see, for example Magoun, 1954). This diffuse projection system appears to be anatomically and functionally different from the specific ascending sensory pathways, even if both are activated by impulses from the same receptors. However, recent anatomical research has made clear that the distinction may not be as sharp as originally assumed, and that certain concepts are in need of revision (as discussed recently by Brodal, 1957, and Rossi and Zanchetti, 1957).

On account of the differences in function and in fibre composition between the cranial nerves, the symptoms which occur when they are affected by disease will vary. The more important symptoms will be described when the individual nerves are dealt with below. Here only some general features will be summarized. With regard to the *somatic efferent cranial nerves*, distinction is made between different types of paralyses or pareses (fig. 4). A *peripheral paralysis* is one due to a damage of the peripheral motor neurons (C, D in fig. 4). If the perikarya are affected (C), a *nuclear paralysis* ensues, if the paralysis is due to an affection of the axons of these perikarya, the efferent fibres (D), the paralysis is referred to as *infra-nuclear*. The motor deficit is identical in the two cases. If not

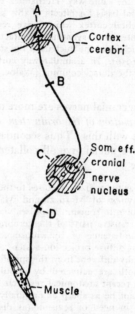

Fig. 4. Diagram explaining the difference between central and peripheral motor paralyses. Explanation in text.

all of the cells or fibres are damaged, there will be an incomplete paralysis (paresis), and there is reduced power on contraction of the muscle. If all cells or fibres are destroyed there is a *complete loss of muscular power* (paralysis), and all movements of the muscles in question are abolished. *Reflex contractions*, correspondingly, are *weakened or abolished*, respectively (for example the corneal reflex, closure of the eyelids on touching

26

the cornea, in a facial palsy). The *tonus of the muscles is reduced* (hypotonia). After some time the affected muscles become *atrophic*. Particularly in nuclear palsies *fasciculation* may occur, i.e. spontaneously appearing twitchings in groups of muscle fibres. These can not be voluntarily suppressed, and are generally assumed to be caused by a state of irritation of the affected peripheral motor neurons. They may, however, be seen also in infranuclear processes.[1]

A paralysis may also be due to a damage to the central motor pathways which mediate impulses to the somatic efferent nuclei. In a paralysis of this type, referred to as *central* or *supranuclear* (A, B, fig. 4), atrophy of the affected muscles will usually be absent. The reflex contractions will be preserved, and frequently they can be elicited more easily than normally. There is no hypotonia, but not infrequently hypertonia. In central paresis the speed of the movements will usually be reduced to a greater degree than one might expect from the commonly moderate reduction in muscular strength, while in peripheral pareses the retardation of the movements appears to correspond to the degree of paresis.

If *sensory tracts or sensory fibres are damaged*, a varying degree of reduced sensibility, e.g. of hearing, will occur, depending upon which nerve or nerves are affected. Reflexes which are elicited on stimulation of receptors innervated by the damaged nerve, will be weakened or abolished. In addition to such *symptoms of deficiency*, *symptoms of irritation* may occur when the sensory fibres are affected by a pathological process, for example paraesthesias in the skin, tinnitus. Occasionally both types of symptoms occur together, for example if a nerve is completely interrupted by a pathological process, which

[1] In the diagnosis of peripheral paralyses electromyography (recording of the electrical activity of the muscles) may be of diagnostic help and of value in considerations of the prognosis. In a completely denervated muscle, no motor unit activity is found. However, very small potentials of a high frequency (fibrillations) may be recorded. When these occur in a muscle, they are a sign that it has lost its motor innervation. When motor unit potentials reappear, this indicates that some motor fibres have grown out and have re-established contact with muscle fibres.

irritates the central ends of the severed nerve fibres. On account of the considerable variations among the cranial nerves with regard to their fibre composition, the sensory symptoms in cranial nerve lesions may vary widely as will be seen from the following account.

In the presentation of the individual cranial nerves to be given below, their anatomy and certain physiological aspects will be dealt with first. Based on these data a brief account of the function of the nerve is given, followed by a survey of the symptomatology in disease processes which may affect the nerve. It can scarcely be overemphasized that a knowledge of anatomy and physiology is a necessary prerequisite for the understanding of the symptoms following diseases and lesions of the cranial nerves.

The Hypoglossal Nerve

Anatomy

The hypoglossal nerve, the 12th cranial nerve, is the motor nerve of the tongue. It is generally considered as being *purely somatic efferent*. The *hypoglossal nucleus* is a longitudinal column of nerve cells of approximately 2 cm. length situated in the medulla oblongata just lateral to the midline and closely underneath the floor of the 4th ventricle (figs. 2 and 3). Here it bulges as the hypoglossal trigone. The nucleus continues a little below the caudal end of the 4th ventricle (fig. 6). The axons of its large multipolar cells run in a ventral and slightly lateral direction and emerge as 10-15 fibre bundles on the ventral surface of the medulla oblongata in the sulcus between the pyramid and the inferior olive (figs. 5 and 6). The bundles fuse and leave the skull in the hypoglossal canal in the occipital bone. The nerve then makes a bend behind the vagus nerve and the internal carotid artery, courses caudally lateral to these structures and then continues in a caudally convex arch to the root of the tongue. A little above the greater horn of the hyoid bone it disappears between the mylohyoid and hyoglossus muscles and splits in the tongue in branches to the intrinsic muscles of the tongue and to the hyoglossus, genioglossus and

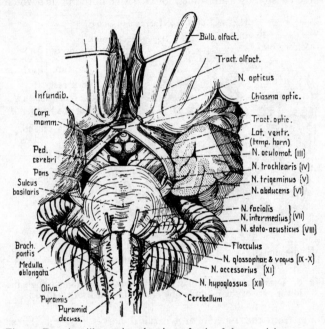

Fig. 5. Drawing illustrating the sites of exit of the cranial nerves on the base of the brain. (From Brodal, 1949.)

styloglossus muscles. According to some authors the nerve also supplies the geniohyoid muscle.

During its peripheral course in the neck the nerve passes below the posterior belly of the digastric muscle and lateral to the internal and external carotid arteries and the branches of the latter. In the tongue the hypoglossal fibres anastomose with branches from the lingual nerve.

29

The somatic efferent fibres of the hypoglossal nerve are joined by some sympathetic (postganglionic) fibres from the superior cervical ganglion of the sympathetic trunk and by some fibres from the nodose ganglion. More important than these anastomoses are some more massive fibre bundles which

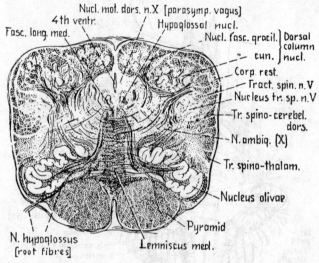

Fig. 6. Drawing of a myelin-stained transverse section through the lower part of the medulla oblongata. (From Brodal, 1949.)

come from the 1st and 2nd cervical nerves (fig. 7). These follow the nerve until the place where it crosses the internal carotid artery. Here they leave it again and descend as the *descending hypoglossal ramus* (ramus descendens hypoglossi), which courses in a caudal direction on the internal carotid artery and the upper part of the common carotid artery. Superficial to the neurovascular sheath this branch unites with the *descending cervical ramus* (ramus descendens cervicalis), which is formed by fibres from the 2nd and 3rd cervical nerves. In this way an arch of fibres, the *ansa hypoglossi*, is formed. It gives off branches to three of the infrahyoid muscles (the

sternohyoid, omohyoid and sternothyroid muscles), while the
fourth of these, the thyrohyoid muscle, is supplied by cervical
fibres which follow the hypoglossal nerve proper beyond the
departure of its descending ramus.

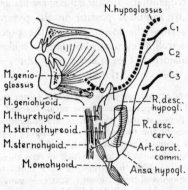

Fig. 7. Diagram of the ansa hypoglossi. (From Brodal, 1948.)

The hypoglossal nucleus is made up of several minor groups of
cells. Experimental studies of the retrograde cellular changes in the
nucleus following extirpation of the various muscles supplied by the
hypoglossal nerve (Barnard, 1940, and others) show that each of these
muscles is supplied by fibres from certain cell groups.

The small nuclei which surround the hypoglossal nucleus (nucl.
intercalatus, nucl. praepositus and nucl. of Roller) have a structure
which differs from that of the main nucleus. Recent experimental
studies have not confirmed the old notion that efferent fibres from
these nuclei join the hypoglossal nerve. A considerable proportion of
their fibres course to the cerebellum (Torvik and Brodal, 1954). The
proximity to the hypoglossal nucleus indicates that there may be
some functional relation between these nuclei and the hypoglossal
nucleus.

The fibres of the hypoglossal nerve are of varying calibre.
Most of them are myelinated. They terminate in the muscles
with characteristic motor end-plates. The innervation of the
tongue by the hypoglossal nerve is strictly ipsilateral. There

31

are good reasons for believing that motor units in the tongue are small.

The cells of the hypoglossal nucleus may be activated by fibres from different sources. *Reflex movements of the tongue* are elicited by impulses entering via other cranial nerves, for example the trigeminal. *Voluntary movements* are assumed to be mediated by impulses passing in the pyramidal tract in fibres coming from the lower part of the precentral gyrus. Anatomical as well as clinical observations make it likely that at least the majority of pyramidal tract fibres acting on the hypoglossal nucleus cross the midline.

In movements of the tongue not only the motor innervation is of importance. The proprioceptive innervation as well must be considered. The demonstration that there are muscle spindles in the intrinsic muscles of the tongue in man (Cooper, 1953) makes clear that the tongue is amply provided with proprioceptive receptors, but it is still an open question along which nerves these impulses are conveyed centrally. Most investigators have failed to find sensory fibres in the hypoglossal nerve, even if scattered ganglion cells occur along its course (Tarkhan and Abd-El Malek, 1950). Some observations may be taken to indicate that the proprioceptive impulses from the tongue pass in the lingual nerve.

Function

The hypoglossal nerve is examined by testing the *mobility* of the tongue and the force exerted by its movements in different directions. Furthermore, one looks for a possible *atrophy* of the musculature of the tongue, and it is noted whether there is *fasciculation* or involuntary movements. Atrophy of the tongue, revealed by reduced volume, is most easily seen when it is unilateral. The tongue is softer and usually flaccid and lacks its tonus. The mucosa of the tongue is more or less wrinkled on the side of atrophy. (This atrophy should be clearly distinguished from the atrophy of the mucous membrane with loss of the lingual papillae which may be seen, for example, in pernicious anaemia.)

Clinical Aspects

When the cells of the hypoglossal nucleus are damaged or destroyed, or when the hypoglossal nerve is interrupted the corresponding half of the tongue will fall victim to atrophy as described above. There will be a *peripheral paralysis* of the hypoglossal nerve. If a patient with a unilateral hypoglossal nerve lesion attempts to protrude his tongue, it will deviate to the affected side because the intact genioglossus muscle (see fig. 7) pulls its half of the tongue forward. Fasciculation is generally taken as a sign that the pathological process has affected the nucleus (and is assumed to be due to abnormal activity in cells in the process of degeneration). The *hypoglossal nerve may be damaged* traumatically or by disease processes in the neck, for example by tumours or diseases in the cervical lymph nodes, or by fractures of the occipital bone (*infranuclear paralysis*). The *hypoglossal nucleus* (*nuclear paralysis*) may be affected in poliomyelitis (bulbar types), usually then together with other motor cranial nerve nuclei. Progressive bulbar palsy frequently affects the hypoglossal nucleus (usually bilaterally). Vascular disorders and inflammations in the medulla oblongata which affect the hypoglossal nerve fibres are usually accompanied by signs of involvement of other structures such as the pyramidal tract (see p. 127 on Wallenberg's syndrome).

A hypoglossal paralysis may occur when the fibres of the pyramidal tract are damaged (*central* or *supranuclear paralysis*). On account of the crossing of the fibres the paralysis will be found on the side contralateral to the lesion. In these cases atrophy of the tongue as well as fasciculation will be absent. A central paralysis of this kind is most frequently met with in capsular hemiplegia (damage to the fibres in the internal capsule). In so-called pseudobulbar palsy, due to progressive degeneration of fibres descending to the motor cranial nerve nuclei, the paralysis is usually bilateral. A unilateral paralysis or paresis of the tongue as a rule is not very invalidating, but when the paralysis is bilateral disturbances of swallowing and speech are apt to occur at an early stage of the disease. Involuntary movements of the tongue may occur in diseases in which such symptoms occur in other muscles as well (chorea, parkinsonism).

Since the infrahyoid muscles are not supplied by fibres of the hypoglossal nerve, they will escape paralysis in lesions which affect the hypoglossal nucleus or are limited to the brain stem. These muscles may be tested by letting the patient press his lower jaw downwards against resistance. The omohyoid muscle in particular can then easily be felt when it contracts, and as a rule can also be seen.

The Accessory Nerve

Anatomy

The 11th cranial nerve, the accessory nerve, is *purely somatic efferent*. It arises as two groups of fibres, a cranial and a spinal, usually referred to as the roots of the nerve. The *cranial root* consists of (special) somatic efferent fibres from the nucleus ambiguus. The fibres leave the medulla oblongata below the lowermost fibres of the vagus nerve and join the fibres of the spinal root (see below). However, they soon again leave this (as a so-called internal ramus) and join the vagus nerve proper above the nodose ganglion (fig. 8). The fibres of the cranial root of the accessory nerve, therefore, may be considered as aberrant vagus fibres, which do not have any functional relation to the accessory nerve proper. This is formed by bundles of somatic efferent fibres which emerge from the lateral funiculus of the spinal cord in the cranial 5-6 cervical segments and together make up the *spinal root*. The fibres ascend within the vertebral canal, fuse with each other and enter the cranial cavity through the foramen magnum. They then join the cranial root, and together the two roots leave the skull through the jugular foramen. The aberrant vagus fibres then depart from the others as the *internal ramus*, and the spinal root fibres continue as the *external ramus*, which alone makes up the accessory nerve in the strict sense. The perikarya of the accessory nerve fibres proper form a longitudinal column of large multipolar nerve cells, situated dorsolaterally in the ventral horn of the cranial 5-6 cervical segments.

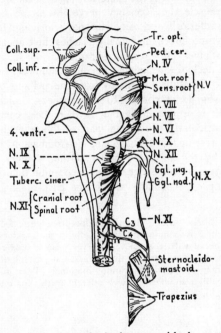

Fig. 8. Dorsolateral view of the brain stem with the rootlets of the 4th-12th cranial nerves. Note the accessory nerve.

Since the embryological origin of the muscles which these fibres supply is debated, there is disagreement as to whether the fibres of the accessory nerve should be considered as special or general somatic efferent.

From the jugular foramen the accessory nerve (the external ramus) descends in close relation to the internal jugular vein

35

(usually posterior, more rarely anterior to it). It is found anterior to the transverse process of the atlas and then enters the sternocleidomastoid muscle on its medial aspect. During its further postero-inferior course the nerve as a rule is embedded in this muscle and gives off branches to it. Approximately at the middle of the posterior aspect of the sternocleidomastoid muscle the accessory nerve leaves the muscle and continues inferiorly and somewhat posteriorly (surrounded by cervical lymph nodes) and finally reaches the trapezius muscle to which it gives off its terminal branches.

In the neck the accessory nerve anastomoses with fibres from the cervical plexus, chiefly from the 3rd and 4th cervical segments (fig. 8). According to some authors, clinical observations make it appear likely that in man these cervical fibres supply particularly the cranial part of the trapezius muscle, while the rest of this and the sternocleidomastoid muscle are supplied by the accessory nerve. Other authors (Monrad-Krohn, 1954; de Jong, 1950) are of the opinion that the cervical fibres supply particularly the lower part of the trapezoid muscle.

Afferent fibres, among them proprioceptive ones, from the two muscles appear to course centrally chiefly in the anastomoses of the accessory nerve with the cervical nerves. Since scattered pseudo-unipolar nerve cells occur in the intracranial part of the accessory nerve, in man as well as in various mammals (Pearson, 1938) this nerve probably also contains some afferent fibres (for references see Brodal, 1948).

Function

The function of the accessory nerve is examined by testing the trapezius and sternocleidomastoid muscles. *Atrophy* is particularly easily observed in the latter. (An atrophy of the sternocleidomastoid muscle, however, does not necessarily indicate a lesion of the accessory nerve. For example, in myotonic dystrophy, atrophy of the sternocleidomastoid muscle is usually an early sign. In this disease it is due to a primary progressive degeneration of the muscle fibres, and is commonly bilateral.) The sternocleidomastoid is tested in a convenient way by letting the standing or sitting patient press his head forwards against resistance, or, if the patient is lying on his back, by letting him lift his head from the pillow. The muscles on either side may then be compared. Paresis or paralysis of the trapezius muscle is more incapacitating than a paresis of the sternocleidomastoid. Thus, elevation of the arm is carried out with reduced force, because the trapezius muscle is important in rotating the scapula around its dorsoventral axis. The scapula will tend to be somewhat lowered, and to have its medial border a little further laterally than normally. The paresis may not be equally marked in the lower and upper parts of the muscle (see above).

Clinical Aspects

Isolated *lesions of the accessory nerve* are rather infrequent. The nucleus of the nerve may be involved for example in poliomyelitis (nuclear paresis). On account of the neighbourhood of the vagus and hypoglossal nerves, lesions of the accessory nerve will frequently affect these two nerves as well, for example in fractures of the base of the skull. In the neck the nerve may be damaged separately in inflammations of the cervical lymph nodes, by tumours or abscesses. When surgical interventions in the posterior triangle of the neck are undertaken, the position of the accessory nerve should be kept in mind.

A lesion of the descending (corticospinal) fibres to the nucleus of the accessory nerve usually produces a paresis or paralysis of the sternocleidomastoid and trapezius muscles. Since at least the majority of these fibres cross the midline, the muscles will be affected contralateral to the lesion (provided this is situated rostral to the pyramidal decussation). There is no clear-cut atrophy (central, supranuclear, paresis).

37

The Vagus Nerve

Anatomy

The 10th cranial nerve, the *vagus nerve*, carries *fibres of all types*. It is predominantly a visceral nerve, and from an embryological point of view it represents the nerves of the 4th, 5th and 6th branchial arches. Its rootlets emerge from the medulla as a series of fibre bundles just dorsal to the inferior olive (figs. 5 and 8). The bundles join and leave the skull in the jugular foramen, where the nerve shows a small swelling, the *jugular ganglion* (ganglion jugulare). Immediately below this the nerve again thickens to form the large, elongated *nodose ganglion* (ganglion nodosum) seen in figs. 8 and 9. The trunk of the vagus nerve then continues in the neck. The efferent fibres proceed without interruption through the ganglia.

The *special somatic efferent fibres* of the vagus nerve come from the *nucleus ambiguus* (nucleus ambiguus, figs. 3 and 6), the *visceral efferent* from the *dorsal motor vagus nucleus* (nucleus motorius dorsalis nervi vagi), also called the parasympathetic vagus nucleus (figs. 3 and 6). The numerous *visceral afferent fibres* have their perikarya in the large *nodose ganglion*, while the *jugular ganglion* (figs. 8 and 9) contains the perikarya of the scanty *somatic afferent fibres*. Before the distribution of the different types of fibres is described, it is appropriate to consider the *peripheral course of the vagus nerve and its branches*.

After the vagus nerve has left the jugular foramen it is found close to the accessory and glossopharyngeal nerves and the internal jugular vein (which all leave the skull through the jugular foramen). The hypoglossal nerve as a rule arches behind these structures to their lateral aspect. The vagus nerve descends in the neck to the upper thoracic aperture and runs between the internal — further down the common — carotid artery medially and the internal jugular vein laterally, enclosed with these in a common sheath of connective tissue. The *right* vagus nerve then descends anterior to the subclavian artery, but

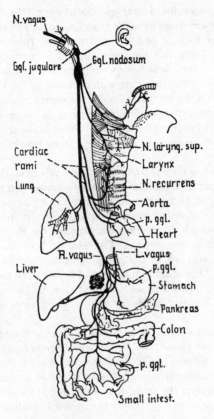

Fig. 9. The chief peripheral branches of the vagus nerve. (From Brodal, 1949, after Grant.)

posterior to the subclavian vein and the superior vena cava and continues on the posterolateral side of the trachea to the posterior aspect of the right main bronchus. It then splits into several anastomosing branches. On the dorsal side of the oesophagus these form a plexus (*plexus oesophagicus*) and anastomose with branches of the left vagus nerve. The terminal branches pierce the diaphragm posterior to the oesophagus and are disseminated over the posterior surface of the stomach where they form a *posterior gastric plexus* (plexus gastricus dorsalis). From this numerous branches (*rami coeliaci*) are given off to the *coeliac ganglion* (ganglion coeliacum). The fibres in these branches pass without interruption through the ganglion and follow the superior mesenteric artery and its arborizations to the small intestine, and to the ascending and transverse colon (*rami intestinales*). Other branches pass to the spleen (*rami lienales*), to the kidneys (*rami renales*) and to the pancreas.

The *trunk of the left vagus nerve* descends from the superior thoracic aperture anterior to the subclavian artery and the aortic arch, and continues posterior to the left main bronchus. On the anterior surface of the oesophagus it splits in anastomosing branches which together with those from the right vagus form the *plexus oesophagicus*. The terminal branches pierce the diaphragm anterior to the oesophagus in the foramen oesophagicum. On the anterior surface of the stomach the branches form a *plexus gastricus ventralis* and give off branches which follow the hepatic artery to the hilum of the liver (*rami hepatici*).

During its *course in the neck and in the chest* the vagus nerve gives off many branches. The *auricular ramus* (ramus auricularis, fig. 9) is a small fibre bundle which takes off at the jugular ganglion, passes through the mastoid canalicus and supplies the dorsal wall of the external auditory meatus and the fundus of the auricle (concha). Where the mastoid canaliculus crosses the facial canal, some fibres from the intermediate nerve enter the auricular ramus. Some other branches from the first part of the vagus should be enumerated. One of these is a *meningeal ramus* (ramus meningicus), which enters the skull in the jugular foramen and supplies the dura mater in the posterior cranial fossa. Other small branches establish anastomoses with the glossopharyngeal nerve and with the superior cervical ganglion of the sympathetic trunk. (As described in the account of the accessory nerve, the internal ramus of this joins the vagus in the jugular foramen.) Furthermore, the vagus nerve gives off *pharyngeal rami* (rami pharyngici) which leave at the nodose ganglion and take a descending and anterior course on the pharynx. They take part in the formation of the *pharyngeal plexus* (plexus pharyngicus) together with branches from the glossopharyngeal nerve and the cervical sympathetic. Somatic efferent fibres from the plexus supply the pharyngeal constrictors (musculi constrictores pharyngici), the soft palate with the levator palati muscle and the muscles of the palatal arches (fig. 9). Sensory fibres from the plexus innervate the mucous membranes of the pharynx and the posterior part of the tongue with the upper surface of the epiglottis.

The *superior laryngeal nerve* (n. laryngicus superior s. cranialis) leaves the trunk of the vagus nerve just below the nodose ganglion and courses in an inferior and a slightly anterior direction on the lateral side of the pharynx (fig. 9). At the greater horn of the hyoid bone it subdivides into an *external ramus*, which carries chiefly somatic efferent fibres to the cricothyroid muscle, and a larger *internal ramus*. The latter enters the larynx through the thyrohyoid membrane immediately below the greater horn of the hyoid bone and is distributed within the larynx. (Before it enters the larynx the nerve produces a ridge in the mucous membrane in the pharynx, the plica nervi laryngici.) The internal ramus supplies the mucous membrane of the larynx down to the vocal cords, and thus is a sensory nerve for the larynx. Electrical stimulation of the nerve in man has shown that it mediates impulses of pain and touch (Ogura and Lam, 1953).

The *recurrent laryngeal nerve* (nervus recurrens, fig. 9), on the other hand, is first and foremost the motor nerve for the larynx. It leaves the trunk of the vagus nerve at a higher level on the right than on the left, because it bends around and behind the subclavian artery on the right, around the aortic arch on the left. Its further course is identical on the two sides. The nerve ascends in the sulcus between the trachea and the oesophagus. Its terminal branch, the *inferior laryngeal nerve* (nervus laryngicus inferior) enters the larynx between the cricoid and thyroid cartilages and splits into a posterior (dorsal) and an anterior (ventral) branch, which innervate the intrinsic laryngeal muscles. (Shortly before the nerve enters the larynx it crosses the inferior thyroid artery, a fact of importance in surgical interventions on the thyroid gland.) The recurrent laryngeal nerve sends branches also to the trachea and oesophagus and some *inferior cardiac rami* (rami cardiaci inferiores) to the heart.

The most important *branches of the vagus nerve to the heart* are, however, the *superior cardiac rami* (rami cardiaci superiores). These leave the vagus nerve between the points of departure of the superior laryngeal nerve and the recurrent nerve and follow the common carotid artery, and on the right side the innominate artery, to the heart. A considerable proportion of these fibres are visceral efferent, and with the inferior cardiac rami they take part in the formation of the *cardiac plexus* (plexus cardiacus). They terminate in synaptical contact with postganglionic (parasympathetic) neurons in the *cardiac ganglia* (ganglii cardiaci). (The sympathetic fibres which are present in the plexus, however, are postganglionic fibres from the cervical sympathetic ganglia.) Other vagus fibres are visceral afferent. Many of these course in a special upper branch of the superior cardiac rami, usually called the *depressor nerve*, because afferent impulses in this nerve produce a lowering of blood pressure. Most of the superior cardiac rami are distributed to the *deep cardiac plexus* (plexus cardiacus profundus) behind the aortic arch just above the bifurcation of the trachea. The left lower branch, which descends more anteriorly, in front of the aortic arch, forms the *superficial cardiac plexus* (plexus cardiacus superficialis) in the concavity of the aortic arch.

The *thoracic part of the vagus nerve* gives off branches to the oesophagus, the bronchi, and the pericardium. The *bronchial rami* (rami bronchiales) are commonly subdivided into anterior and posterior, and form (together with postganglionic sympathetic fibres) *anterior and posterior pulmonary plexuses* (plexus pulmonalis ventralis et dorsalis) which surround the bronchi. These plexuses continue along the branches of the bronchial tree into the lung. The postganglionic neurons which are found in the plexuses finally transmit the visceral efferent impulses to the glands and the smooth muscles of the air passages.

The terminal branches of the vagus in the abdomen have been dealt with above.

As has been mentioned, the *somatic efferent fibres of the vagus nerve* have their perikarya in the *nucleus ambiguus*. This nucleus forms a longitudinal column, about 16 mm. long, in the ventrolateral part of the medulla (figs. 3 and 6) and is made up of large multipolar nerve cells. Rostrally it reaches almost to the facial nucleus. From the nucleus the fibres pass in a dorsally directed arch before they turn ventrally (see fig. 2 and the course of the fibres of the facial nerve). By way of the pharyngeal rami they innervate the striated musculature of the palate and pharynx, and through the recurrent and the superior laryngeal nerves the muscles of the larynx.

Experimental studies indicate that the different groups of muscles supplied by the vagus nerve receive their fibres from different parts of the nucleus ambiguus (Getz and Sirnes, 1949). Even the various intrinsic laryngeal muscles appear to be 'represented' in definite parts of the nucleus (Szentágothai, 1943a). The fibres to the larynx largely pass via the cranial root of the accessory nerve (DuBois and Foley, 1936). The rostralmost part of the nucleus ambiguus gives origin to the somatic efferent fibres of the glossopharyngeal nerve (see p. 50). The cortical innervation of the nucleus ambiguus appears to be bilateral, and is assumed to take place through corticobulbar fibres which follow the pyramidal tract (see p. 24).

The *visceral efferent fibres* in the vagus nerve come from the columnar *dorsal motor (parasympathetic) nucleus of the vagus*. This is found underneath the floor of the 4th ventricle, just lateral to the hypoglossal nucleus (figs. 3 and 6) and is made up of small multipolar nerve cells. Their axons course in a ventral direction to the rootlets of the nerve. Visceral efferent fibres are found in the branches of the vagus nerve to the oesophagus, trachea, bronchi, heart, stomach and intestines, pancreas, spleen and liver, but in addition a smaller number run in the superior laryngeal nerve to supply the glands of the larynx. These visceral efferent fibres are preganglionic and, as mentioned previously, establish synaptical contact with autonomic nerve cells in the various plexuses and ganglia which have been mentioned above. In the stomach and the intestines the post-ganglionic perikarya are found in the submucous and myenteric plexuses.

According to the experimental studies of Getz and Sirnes (1949) the fibres to the various organs arise from different regions of the dorsal motor nucleus of the vagus, those to the lungs in the rostral part, those to the heart and oesophagus in the caudal half. In this connexion it is of interest that in animals as well as in man (Olszewski and Baxter, 1954) the nucleus is composed of cells of different types, and that cells of each type are collected predominantly in certain regions of the nucleus. This is probably a morphological feature of functional importance.

The numerous *visceral afferent vagus fibres* have their perikarya in the nodose ganglion (DuBois and Foley, 1937). They mediate afferent impulses from the visceral organs which are supplied by the vagus as well as taste impulses from the posterior part of the tongue (see p. 72). In the medulla the central processes of the ganglion cells turn in a caudal direction. These longitudinally running fibres together make up the *solitary tract* (tractus solitarius), a distinct fibre bundle which can easily be recognized in myelin sheath stained sections. It can be traced from the caudal end of the medulla almost to the level of the facial nucleus. The terminal branches of these fibres and their collaterals establish synaptical contact with nerve cells which surround the solitary tract and constitute the *nucleus of the solitary tract* (nucleus tractus solitarii, figs. 3 and 13). The cells of this nucleus, which are sensory neurons of the second order, give off axons which ascend in the brain stem. At least some of them reach the thalamus (nucleus lateralis) and thus form a link in the pathways which mediate visceral afferent impulses to higher levels (see the pathways of taste, p. 72 ff. and fig. 14).

In addition to visceral afferent fibres of the vagus nerve, similar fibres of the glossopharyngeal and intermediate nerves also take part

44

in the formation of the solitary tract. Experimental studies (Torvik, 1956; and others) have shown that the latter fibres enter the tract rostral to the vagus fibres, those of the intermediate nerve most rostrally. In man the same arrangement is found (Schwartz, Roulhac, Lam and O'Leary, 1951). The fibres end in the same order in the nucleus of the solitary tract. (Even some trigeminal fibres end in this nucleus as shown by Torvik, 1956.)

Some authors in addition to the nucleus of the solitary tract describe a *dorsal sensory vagus nucleus*, which is situated dorsomedial to the former. Others consider it to be part of the nucleus of the solitary tract, with which it is continuous. There are some structural differences between the two nuclei, which may indicate that they are functionally dissimilar.

The *somatic afferent vagus fibres* have their perikarya in the jugular ganglion (DuBois and Foley, 1937). The majority of these fibres pass in the auricular ramus (fig. 9) which is purely sensory. Centrally they join the afferent fibres of the trigeminal nerve and take a corresponding course (see p. 89). Normal anatomical as well as experimental studies in animals (Ingram and Dawkins, 1945, and others) have demonstrated that these fibres terminate principally in the nucleus of the spinal trigeminal tract and are distributed to its most dorsal part. This nucleus is the terminal station of fibres which transmit impulses of pain and temperature from the head (see p. 89 ff.). Following a medullary tractotomy (p. 91), however, the sense of pain is lost not only in those regions which are supplied by the trigeminal nerve and the auricular ramus of the vagus nerve, but also in the posterior part of the tongue and in the pharynx (Brodal, 1947a; Falconer, 1949). Therefore, vagus (and glossopharyngeal) fibres which transmit impulses from these regions must be assumed to end in the nucleus of the spinal trigeminal tract.[1] The central course of the fibres from this nucleus are dealt with in the section on the trigeminal nerve.

[1] On an embryological basis all sensory impulses from the pharynx and posterior part of the tongue will have to be classified as visceral. However, their relation to the somatic afferent trigeminal nucleus makes it appear doubtful if this is rational. The fact that pain impulses from the pharynx are distinctly perceived and can be fairly well localized by the individual, indicates close relations to somatic sensibility. This is only one of many examples which show that the borders between 'somatic' and 'visceral' are diffuse.

The vagus nerve contains fibres of varying diameters and a considerable number of unmyelinated fibres. Below the nodose ganglion 67-77 per cent of the fibres are unmyelinated in the cat (Foley and DuBois, 1937). The thicker fibres which are found here are presumably in part somatic efferent fibres to the laryngeal muscles which run in the recurrent nerve. However, since not all thicker fibres degenerate following a transection of the vagus nerve central to its ganglion, some of them must be afferent, presumably chiefly sensory fibres from the larynx. The fact that following such operations 30 per cent of the fibres in the predominantly sensory superior laryngeal nerve are intact, against 3 per cent in the recurrent nerve (Brocklehurst and Edgeworth, 1940) supports this assumption. In man the superior laryngeal nerve contains some 15,000 fibres, and most of them are myelinated. Somewhat more than 30 per cent of the fibres are thick, 10-15 µ (Ogura and Lam, 1953).

Function

On account of its wide distribution and its composition of fibres of all types, the *vagus nerve is concerned with many functions*.

Most simple to assess are *motor deficiency symptoms*, due to damage to the somatic efferent fibres. A peripheral damage to the vagus nerve will be followed by a *paralysis of the laryngeal muscles* on the same side and a varying degree of *paresis of the pharynx*. On attempts to move the velum palati and the pharynx (for example when the patient is asked to say 'ah') the raphes of the soft palate and pharynx will deviate to the normal side. The velum will be elevated less on the affected side on account of the paresis of the levator palati muscle. The same is seen when a contraction is elicited reflexly by touching the palate or the pharynx (palatal reflex, pharyngeal reflex). Speech and particularly swallowing are made difficult. Food and especially drinks are apt to enter the nasopharynx in the act of swallowing, because the closure of the nasopharynx from the oropharynx by the soft palate is deficient. *Paresis or paralysis of the laryngeal muscles* may occur in lesions of the vagus nerve or of the nucleus ambiguus but is far more commonly seen as a consequence of lesions of the recurrent nerve. In the latter case, there will not be other symptoms from the vagus nerve. Since laryngoscopy permits an accurate determination of the condition of the laryngeal muscles, this examination should be undertaken whenever there may be suspicion of a lesion of the vagus nerve, even if there are not clear-cut changes of the patient's voice (hoarseness or other aberrations). According to the degree of the damage to the nerve, varying degrees of paralysis of the vocal apparatus may occur. In a recurrent nerve palsy it is common that the muscles which separate the vocal cords and open the rima glottidis (the so-called abductor muscles, chiefly the posterior crico-arytaenoid muscle) suffer first (Semon's law). The vocal cord on the affected side will then move towards the midline. When the recurrent nerve paralysis on one side is complete, the vocal cord on this side will be in an abducted position (cadaveric position). After some time the patient learns how to adapt the innervation of the muscles on the non-affected side, so that the vocal cords again may be brought into contact, and the hoarseness which was originally present on account of the paresis, again disappears. Bilateral complete paralysis of the recurrent nerves is followed by aphonia (loss of the voice) since both vocal cords are in the abducted position.

Why the abductor muscles are usually affected first in a developing paralysis of the recurrent nerve is unknown. It has been assumed that the nerve fibres to these muscles are particularly vulnerable, or that the fibres may be collected in a bundle which is more exposed to damage than the other fibres. The fibres to the abductor muscles have been assumed to pass in the posterior branch of the inferior laryngeal nerve. An analysis of the arrangement of the fibres of this nerve in man (Sunderland and Swaney, 1952) has shown, however, that fibres to the different groups of laryngeal muscles intermingle in their course. It is of interest that in some cases, in which a unilateral vocal cord paralysis has been suspected, electromyographic investigations have shown the impaired mobility of the cords to be due to an ankylosis in the crico-arytaenoid joints (Weddell, Feinstein and Pattle, 1944).

Sensory deficiency symptoms in lesions of the vagus nerve will manifest themselves as a reduced or abolished sensibility in the pharynx and larynx, and sometimes in the concha of the auricle. With regard to the pharynx and the ear, an intact glossopharyngeal nerve may reduce or mask the loss of the vagal innervation. Lesions which produce an *irritation* of the superior laryngeal nerve may cause attacks of coughing and other reflex phenomena, elicited from the larynx, such as excessive production of mucus. Neuralgias of the superior laryngeal nerve occur.

In the *autonomic sphere*, affections of the vagus nerve may produce a multitude of changes, which, however, are usually difficult to ascertain. An *interruption of the visceral efferent fibres* may cause reduction of secretion and peristalsis in the stomach and intestines, reduced secretion of mucus and dilatation of the bronchi. On account of the intermingling of fibres from the right and left vagus nerves and because the peripheral, postganglionic neurons in the autonomic plexus appear to have some capacity to function independently of the central nervous system, the alterations in the autonomic sphere following damage to the vagus nerve will not be very marked or of great practical importance. This is substantiated in surgical sections of the nerve (vagotomy). Interruption of the nerve, particularly if it is bilateral, may result in an increased heart rate. The *visceral afferent vagus fibres* chiefly play a role in a number of reflexes. Lesions which produce an irritation of the nerve may elicit symptoms from visceral efferent fibres (increased secretion and peristalsis in the stomach and the intestines, lowering of the heart rate, constriction of the respiratory passages with increased secretion of mucus) or from the visceral afferent fibres (retching, changes in blood pressure, reflex alterations of the secretion of mucus in the airways, secretion of gastric juice, etc.).

Clinical Aspects

The causes of lesions of the vagus nerve during its course are many. The nerve may suffer in various processes in the neck, such as tumours or inflammations in the cervical lymph nodes, aneurysms of the internal carotid artery, open traumatic injuries. The larger branches may also be involved alone, a damage to the recurrent nerve being the most important of such lesions. On account of the topography of this nerve paralysis of the vocal cords may occur not only when the trunk of the vagus nerve is affected, but also in other instances, as for example in aneurysms on the aortic arch (left recurrent nerve), aneurysms on the subclavian artery (right recurrent nerve), enlargement of the tracheo-bronchial lymph nodes (in tuberculosis, lymphogranulomatosis, leukaemia), tumours in the mediastinum. The recurrent nerve may also be injured in operations on the thyroid gland. In some instances no particular cause can be found. It is common then to speak of an idiopathic paralysis of the recurrent nerve. It has been suggested that an inflammation of the nerve may be responsible.

Symptoms due to involvement of the somatic efferent vagus fibres, paralysis of the pharynx and larynx, may be seen not only in lesions of the vagus nerve but also when *disease processes affect the perikarya of the fibres in the nucleus ambiguus*, for example in poliomyelitis, progressive bulbar palsy (nuclear paralysis). Tumours, inflammations and vascular disorders in the medulla, such as a thrombosis of the inferior posterior cerebellar artery (see Wallenberg's syndrome, p. 127), in addition to symptoms from the vagus nerve will usually give evidence of damage to other nuclei and tracts as well. Bilateral affections of the somatic efferent vagus fibres as a rule produce severe difficulties in deglutition, which are commonly an important contributing factor in the fatal issue of bilateral affections of the vagus. *Supranuclear vagus paralyses* are seen only in bilateral affections of the corticobulbar fibres, for example in pseudobulbar palsy, since the nucleus ambiguus receives a bilateral cortical innervation (see p. 43). A particular type of paralysis of branches of the vagus nerve is seen after diphtheria of the throat. The local action of the spreading diphtheria toxin on the nerve fibres in the soft palate produces a paresis or paralysis of the soft palate (see Fisher and Adams, 1956), but other nerves may also be affected. Also in botulism pareses of muscles in the pharynx and larynx on a toxic basis occur.

The Glossopharyngeal Nerve

Anatomy

The 9th cranial nerve, the glossopharyngeal, is closely related
to the vagus nerve. It is formed by 5-6 small fibre bundles
which emerge from the medulla oblongata immediately rostral
to the vagus fibres (figs. 5 and 8). The nerve courses in a
ventral direction and leaves the skull in the anteromedial part
of the jugular foramen. It then descends in an arch with its
convexity inferoposteriorly to the base of the tongue where it
splits into its terminal branches. It lies on the lateral wall of
the pharynx, but lateral to the internal carotid artery, and at
the base of the tongue it turns in a medially directed bend over
the lateral side of the stylopharyngeus muscle. Like the vagus
nerve the glossopharyngeal has two sensory ganglia. The
small *superior ganglion* (ganglion superius) is situated as a small
swelling of the nerve in the jugular foramen, the somewhat
larger *petrosal ganglion* (ganglion petrosum) is found in a small
fossa (fossula petrosa) just outside the jugular foramen. Both
ganglia are made up of pseudounipolar ganglion cells.

The glossopharyngeal nerve carries the same types of fibres
as the vagus nerve. The *somatic efferent fibres* arise in the
rostral part of the *nucleus ambiguus*, the *visceral efferent ones*
appear to be derived from a small cell group, the *inferior
salivatory nucleus* (nucleus salivatorius inferior), which is
situated immediately rostral to the dorsal motor (parasympathetic) vagus nucleus (fig. 3). These fibres are preganglionic
parasympathetic. *Visceral afferent fibres*, which have their
perikarya in the petrosal ganglion, join the solitary tract in its
rostral part and end at corresponding levels in the nucleus of
the solitary tract (fig. 14). Some of these fibres are special
visceral afferent fibres from taste buds in the tongue. Finally,
as mentioned in the account of the vagus nerve, the glossopharyngeal nerve contains some fibres which end in the nucleus
of the spinal trigeminal tract, and accordingly should be
grouped as *somatic afferent*.

As its name indicates, the glossopharyngeal nerve supplies first and foremost the tongue and the pharynx. Its terminal branches in the tongue (*rami linguales*) are distributed to the mucous membrane on the posterior third of the tongue and the vallate papillae. These branches, in addition to afferent fibres from the mucosa, among them taste fibres, contain also visceral efferent fibres to the small salivary glands in the area of innervation. *Pharyngeal branches* (rami pharyngici) take off from the trunk of the nerve lateral to the internal carotid artery and supply the pharyngeal wall. Together with fibres from the vagus and sympathetic fibres they make up the *pharyngeal plexus* (plexus pharyngicus). It is an open question to what extent fibres from the vagus and the glossopharyngeal nerves supply particular regions of the pharynx, but the vagus fibres appear to be quantitatively most important. The glossopharyngeal fibres to the pharynx are of different kinds. Somatic efferent fibres innervate the striated musculature of the pharynx, visceral efferent (secretory) fibres supply the glands in the mucosa (postganglionic neurons in this), and finally there are visceral afferent fibres which correspond to those of the vagus nerve.

In addition to the lingual and pharyngeal branches the glossopharyngeal nerve gives off some smaller branches. A *stylopharyngeal branch* (ramus stylopharyngicus) innervates the muscle of the same name, and *tonsillar branches* (rami tonsillares) supply the tonsil and palatal arches. By means of an anastomosis with the auricular ramus of the vagus nerve somatic afferent glossopharyngeal fibres take part in the innervation of the concha of the auricle. A particular branch is the *tympanic nerve* (nervus tympanicus, fig. 17). It leaves the petrosal ganglion and enters the tympanic cavity through a small bony channel (canaliculus tympanicus inferior). It ascends on the promontorium of the tympanic cavity (by way of the caroticotympanic nerves it here receives sympathetic fibres from the plexus on the internal carotid artery) and enters the cranial cavity through a small channel in the tegmen of the tympanic cavity (canalicus tympanicus superior). Then the nerve courses as the *lesser superficial petrosal nerve* (nervus petrosus superficialis minor, fig. 17) anteriorly on the pyramid of the temporal bone and again leaves the cranial cavity (through the sphenopetrosal fissure) to end in the parasympathetic *otic ganglion* (ganglion oticum), situated just below the oval foramen (p. 87).

The tympanic nerve and its continuation, the lesser superficial petrosal nerve, carry chiefly visceral efferent fibres, assumed to come from the inferior salivatory nucleus. In the otic ganglion the fibres establish synaptical contact with postganglionic neurons. The axons of these enter the auriculotemporal nerve (a branch of the trigeminal nerve) and supply the parotid gland with secretory fibres (fig. 17). Sensory fibres of the tympanic nerve innervate the mucous membranes of the tympanic cavity and the Eustachian tube.

Finally a small branch of the glossopharyngeal nerve, the so-called *nerve of the carotid sinus* or ramus caroticus nervi glossopharyngici, deserves mention. It leaves the trunk of the nerve (less frequently the pharyngeal rami) and runs to the bifurcation of the common carotid artery. Here it innervates the walls of the carotid sinus (Boyd, 1937). Frequently fibres can also be traced to the carotid body. This nerve commonly has small anastomoses with the vagus nerve. Its fibres end chiefly in the thick adventitia of the carotid sinus, to a small extent only in its thin tunica media, and are, at least predominantly, afferent. These fibres form the afferent link in the arc of the carotid sinus reflex, which is elicited on stimulation of mechanoreceptors in the sinus, and of the reflexes elicited on stimulation of the chemoreceptors in the carotid body.

Function and Clinical Aspects

From a functional point of view the glossopharyngeal nerve is closely related to the vagus nerve. Lesions of the nerve will result in loss of taste on the posterior third of the tongue, in a certain loss of muscular power in the pharynx and reduced sensibility in the pharynx, on the palatal arches and in the concha of the auricle. Reduction of the secretion of the parotid gland may be expected. On account of the ample intermingling of fibres of the glossopharyngeal and vagus nerves in the pharyngeal plexus, it will be difficult to diagnose clinically a pure glossopharyngeal nerve lesion. (On account of their close topographical relations, it is common to find both these nerves affected simultaneously, in lesions of the nerves as well as in lesions of their nuclei.) The most decisive criterion of an affection of the glossopharyngeal nerve is the determination of loss of taste in the posterior third of the tongue. This, however, is difficult when the usual tests for taste sensibility are used, but can be made with the galvanic test (see Monrad-Krohn, 1954). A *glossopharyngeal neuralgia*, pain in the regions of distribution of the nerve, occurring in paroxysms, is occasionally met with. In some cases surgical interruption of the nerve central to its ganglia has given relief.

The Stato-acoustic Nerve

Anatomy

The 8th cranial nerve was formerly frequently named the *acoustic nerve*. Since it actually is made up of two functionally different components, the *vestibular nerve* and the *cochlear nerve*, it is now preferentially referred to as the stato-acoustic nerve, the nerve of equilibrium and hearing. Both components are special somatic afferent and conduct impulses centrally from the apparatus of equilibrium and the acoustic organ, respectively, in the inner ear. They leave the brain stem together on the lateral surface of the medulla, just beneath the caudal border of the pons (figs. 5 and 8), the vestibular nerve being ventral to the cochlear. Some bundles of the latter nerve emerge dorsal to the restiform body. Ventral to the vestibular nerve the facial and intermediate nerves leave the brain stem.

From the lateral surface of the brain stem the stato-acoustic nerve (together with the facial and intermediate nerves) enters the internal auditory meatus (porus acusticus internus) and can be followed as a large fibre bundle to its bottom. Here the nerve splits into different branches which supply various divisions of the membraneous labyrinth. It will be appropriate to describe the two parts of the stato-acoustic nerve separately.

The Vestibular Nerve

The special somatic afferent fibres of the nerve are processes of bipolar ganglion cells. These are situated in the bottom of the internal auditory meatus where they form the *vestibular ganglion* (ganglion vestibuli). The central processes of these cells make up the vestibular nerve. The peripheral ones course as several smaller bundles to the different parts of the vestibular apparatus: the cristae of the three semicircular ducts, the maculae of the utricle and the saccule.[1]

The central processes of the vestibular ganglion cells which enter the brain stem course between the restiform body dorsally and the nucleus of the spinal trigeminal tract ventrally. Most of them dichotomize in an ascending and a descending branch. They give off collaterals to and finally end in the four vestibular nuclei. These are situated immediately underneath the floor of the fourth ventricle, largely in its lateral recess (figs. 3, 10 and 13). Some of the descending fibres take part in the formation of a distinct fibre bundle, the *descending or spinal vestibular root* (radix descendens s. spinalis n. vestibuli) and end in the *descending or spinal vestibular nucleus* (nucleus vestibularis descendens s. spinalis, fig. 10). The other vestibular nuclei are the *medial vestibular nucleus* (nucleus vestibularis medialis s. triangularis, Schwalbe), the *superior vestibular nucleus* (nucleus vestibularis superior, Bechterew) and the *lateral vestibular nucleus* (nucleus vestibularis lateralis,

[1] According to recent investigations the sacculus appears to differ functionally from the utriculus and, at least in part, to serve as a receptor for slow mechanical vibrations. Anastomoses exist between the cochlear and vestibular nerve, but their significance is not clearly understood (see Shute, 1951).

Deiters). The latter is characterized by containing many large multipolar cells.[1]

The morphological subdivision of the vestibular nuclei into different parts leads one to assume that the various nuclei differ with regard to their afferent and efferent fibre connexions, and thus are not functionally equivalent. The study of these problems meets with many difficulties, and many questions in their detailed anatomy are still open. Summarizing it may be stated that the efferent fibres from the vestibular nuclei are so arranged as to be able to influence chiefly three other regions of the central nervous system: the cerebellum, the spinal cord and the nuclei of the extrinsic muscles of the eye (fig. 10). Furthermore, impulses from the vestibular apparatus reach the cerebral cortex. It will suffice here with a broad outline of the pathways taken by the impulses leaving the vestibular nuclei.

Cerebellar afferent fibres terminate in the phylogenetically oldest part of the cerebellum, the flocculonodular lobe (Dow, 1936). They are derived chiefly from the medial and descending vestibular nuclei (Brodal and Torvik, 1957). Primary vestibular fibres end in the same parts of the cerebellum and the uvula (Brodal and Høivik, 1964).

Most of the *fibres to the spinal cord* come from the lateral vestibular nucleus of Deiters and make up the vestibulospinal tract which descends in the homolateral ventrolateral funiculus to the sacral segments. Its fibres, which originate in a somatotopic manner from the nucleus of Deiters (Pompeiano and Brodal, 1957a), end in the ventral horn of the cord but do not establish contact with motoneurons (Nyberg-Hansen and Mascitti, 1964). Other fibres derived from the medial vestibular nuclei descend in the medial longitudinal fasciculus and are present only in the cervical segment of the cord (Nyberg-Hansen, 1964).

The secondary *vestibular fibres to the nuclei of the extrinsic eye muscles* make up a considerable part of the phylogenetically old *medial*

[1] A closer analysis reveals that in addition to the four classical nuclei the vestibular complex contains certain minor cell groups, which to some extent have their particular fibre connexions (Brodal and Pompeiano, 1957a). Furthermore, primary vestibular fibres do not supply all regions of the four principal vestibular nuclei. For example, only the ventral part of the lateral nucleus of Deiters receives such fibres (Walberg, Bowsher and Brodal, 1958). For a recent account on the connexions and functional aspects of the vestibular nuclei see the monograph of Brodal, Pompeiano and Walberg (1962).

longitudinal bundle (fasciculus longitudinalis medialis). This can be followed as a distinct bundle ventral to the ventricular system from the medulla to the mesencephalon (figs. 6, 10 and 13). It continues in the ventral funiculus of the cord as the *sulcomarginal fasciculus*.

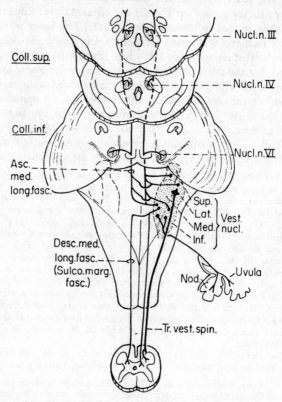

Fig. 10. Simplified diagram of the principal efferent connexions of the vestibular nuclei according to recent studies.

The composition of the medial longitudinal bundle is very complex. In addition to descending fibres from two small nuclei in the mesencephalon, it contains ascending fibres from all four vestibular nuclei. (For recent accounts see the papers of Brodal and Pompeiano, 1957b; Pompeiano and Brodal, 1957a; and Pompeiano and Walberg, 1957.)

Some of the latter fibres cross the midline. Some ascend, others descend, still others dichotomize in an ascending and a descending branch (fig. 10). In spite of this, there seems to be a definite order in the arrangement. Thus the superior nucleus appears to send all its fibres in a rostral direction (Buchanan, 1937, and others). A considerable proportion of the ascending secondary vestibular fibres end in the somatic efferent nuclei of the abducent, trochlear and oculomotor nerves which supply the extrinsic eye muscles, and thus mediate vestibular impulses which induce changes in the position of the eyes (see below). For a recent study see Carpenter and McMasters (1963).

There is physiological evidence that impulses from the vestibular nuclei reach the cerebral cortex, but the fibre connexions utilized by these impulses are insufficiently known (see Brodal, Pompeiano and Walberg, 1962, for a recent account).

Recently an *efferent* component has been found in the vestibular nerve. Its fibres appear to be derived from the lateral nucleus of Deiters and to end on the vestibular receptor cells (see Gacek, 1960).

The *vestibular nerve* mediates impulses from the cristae of the semicircular ducts and from the maculae of the utriculus and sacculus. In a simplified fashion it is common to distinguish between a *kinetic labyrinth*, the semicircular ducts, and a *static labyrinth*, the utriculus (and presumably in part also the sacculus, see Szentágothai, 1952). The adequate stimuli for the semicircular ducts are currents in the endolymph which arise on movements of the head. The receptor (hair) cells in the cristae will be stimulated when the hairs and the gelatinous cupula are displaced in the direction of the current. Since the semicircular ducts are arranged in three planes, perpendicular to each other, a movement of the head in any direction will elicit currents in the endolymph and consequently impulses in the nerve fibres leading in a central direction from the ducts. The adequate stimulus to the sensory cells of the maculae appears to be the displacement of the gelatinous otolithic membrane with its otoliths (statoliths) which occurs when the position of the head is altered. Like the cristae, also the maculae react on movements of the head (linear acceleration) although to a lesser degree. Their chief function, however, appears to be the recording of changes in position of the head.

Electrical recording of action potentials from single nerve fibres of individual semicircular ducts in selachians (Löwenstein and Sand, 1940) confirms that the notion of the mode of reaction of the ducts to movements in different directions is correct. Furthermore, the spontaneous activity which is present when the cristae are not stimulated, increases on movements in one direction, but is depressed by movements in the opposite direction. The co-operation between the various semicircular ducts represents a finely co-ordinated integration. Recordings from the vestibular nuclei (Adrian, 1943) show that impulses from different parts of the receptor organ activate different cell groups in the vestibular nuclei (see also Gernandt, 1959).

Function

The complex patterns of nervous impulses which are conveyed in a central direction when the position of the head is changed or it is moved act, first and foremost, in initiating some important *reflexes*. As concerns *movements of the eyes* the semicircular ducts are the most important. They secure a finely differentiated innervation of the individual extrinsic eye muscles, which enables us to keep our gaze fixed on an object even if we are moving. The static labyrinth, also, is of some importance for movements of the eyes, but plays a greater role in the reflex changes in the *tonus of the muscles of the body*. The tonic labyrinthine reflexes produce appropriate changes in muscle tone, according to the position of the head.[1] The most important connexions in the arcs of these reflexes are the medial longitudinal bundle and the connexions from the vestibular nuclei to the spinal cord, respectively. The details in the arcs of these reflexes are not yet known. Obviously rather complex fibre connexions and impulse patterns are involved. However, sufficient is known to be of practical use.

The *examination of the function of the vestibular nerve* is based on testing reflexes such as those described above. In the common clinical tests the functions of the static and kinetic labyrinth cannot be kept apart (and as mentioned above, they

[1] The semicircular ducts are, however, also involved in these reflexes (see Szentágothai, 1952) as is learnt from clinical tests (see below).

appear to interact). The most commonly employed test method is to examine the occurrence of nystagmus, spontaneous or artificially induced.

The term *nystagmus* is used for conjugate rhythmic movements of the eyes, when the eyeballs are turned rapidly in one direction and return more slowly to their starting position. In spite of the slow phase being the active, the rapid one only a passive returning movement, for practical reasons the direction of the nystagmus is indicated with reference to its rapid phase. Many types of nystagmus occur, but only some of them will be considered here. Nystagmus may be *spontaneous*, i.e. it is present also when the head is kept still.[1] This is always pathological.[2] Nystagmus may be induced by *optic stimuli* (optokinetic nystagmus, see p. 117). It may also be *produced experimentally by stimulating the semicircular ducts* artificially in various ways. In these tests, currents are produced in the endolymph, and this elicits nystagmus movements in a particular direction, depending on which of the ducts are being stimulated. Experimentally a very close correlation has been demonstrated between stimulation of particular ducts and movements in a certain direction, and corresponding observations can be made clinically. In the *rotatory test* the patient is turned around his own axis with his head kept in a certain position, the turning being standardized with regard to its duration and speed. When the turning is suddenly stopped, a nystagmus is observed due to the current in the endolymph, which, on account of the inertia of the fluid, will continue to stream for a while in the direction in which the rotation took place. By this procedure both labyrinths are tested simultaneously. In the *caloric test* instillation of cold or warm water in one external auditory meatus produces currents in the endolymph which elicit nystagmus. In this test each labyrinth is tested separately. Together with the nystagmus,

[1] A spontaneous nystagmus may be present only when the head is kept in a certain position, or it may change in intensity according to the position in which the head is kept (positional nystagmus).
[2] However, spontaneous nystagmus may be seen as a congenital anomaly which has no clinical significance.

changes in muscular tonus occur (see p. 58) such that the patient tends to fall to one side. If the patient tries to point with his eyes closed, his arm will deviate from the correct direction. The direction of falling and of past pointing is opposite to the direction of the nystagmus, i.e. it corresponds to the direction of the *active* phase of the nystagmus.[1]

Clinical Aspects

If the function of the labyrinth on one side is impaired the nystagmus induced by caloric stimulation on this side will have a shorter duration than when the labyrinth on the normal side is stimulated. Similarly, the tendency of falling and of past pointing will be diminished. Such abberations in the normal reactions may be seen in *diseases of the labyrinth*, but also in *lesions of the vestibular nerve*, most commonly as symptoms in so-called acoustic nerve tumours, neurinoma of the 8th cranial nerve (see p. 77).

Affections of the vestibular nuclei and the central vestibular pathways may likewise give rise to symptoms (central nystagmus). In addition to spontaneous nystagmus of different kinds, many variations in the reaction to the vestibular tests may be seen. 'Central nystagmus' is most frequently found in disseminated sclerosis, where it has been assumed to be due to demyelinating foci in the vestibular nuclei or in the medial longitudinal bundle. It may also occur following head injuries. In diseases of the vestibular apparatus or its central connexions dizziness (vertigo) is a common symptom. Also lesions of the cerebral cortex in the terminal area of the vestibular pathways may be followed by vertigo.

The Cochlear Nerve

The perikarya of the special somatic afferent fibres of the cochlear nerve are bipolar ganglion cells which together make

[1] Objective recording of the eye movements in nystagmus is possible by means of electronystagmography (see Aschan, 1956). This method has proved useful in clinical practice.

up the *spiral ganglion* (ganglion spirale). This is situated in the long spiral canal of the cochlea. The peripheral processes of the ganglion cells end around the hair cells of the organ of Corti, the central processes join and form smaller bundles which run towards the base of the cochlea. Through a series of small holes, arranged as a spiral (tractus spiralis foraminosus) they enter the fundus of the internal auditory meatus where they fuse to form the cochlear nerve. In the deeper part of the meatus this is situated in front of the vestibular nerve and below (caudal to) the facial nerve.

As mentioned above the fibres of the cochlear nerve enter the medulla dorsal to and to some extent lateroventral to the restiform body. The fibres terminate in the *dorsal and ventral cochlear nuclei* (nucleus dorsalis et ventralis nervi cochleae). The dorsal nucleus produces the so-called acoustic tubercle (tuberculum acusticum) on the dorsal aspect of the restiform body, the ventral nucleus lies lateral to the restiform body and fuses with the former. The structure of the two nuclei is different. Many of the entering fibres of the acoustic nerve bifurcate into two branches, one to each of the cochlear nuclei. The cells in these give off axons which transmit the impulses centrally. These connexions are rather complicated. In a very simplified way they may be outlined as follows (fig. 11). The pathways mediating conscious perception of sound ascend in the brain stem in the lateral fillet or lemniscus (lemniscus lateralis) and have relay stations in the inferior colliculus and the medial geniculate body (corpus geniculatum mediale). From the latter nucleus the last link in the pathway runs as fibres to the (primary) acoustic cortical area in the superior temporal gyrus. The connexions are crossed and uncrossed. The cortical regions which surround the primary acoustic cortex appear to be essential for the interpretation of acoustic impulses and to represent a secondary acoustic area.

The fibres from the ventral cochlear nucleus turn in a ventral direction and to a large extent cross to the opposite side (fig. 11). The crossing fibres make up the trapezoid body. Some of these secondary sensory fibres terminate in the superior olive (nucleus olivaris superior) on both sides (Stotler, 1953) or in small nuclei embedded in the trapezoid body. Fibres from these nuclei join those which course without interruption to the lateral lemniscus. Also among the fibres of the lateral lemniscus small cell groups are present.

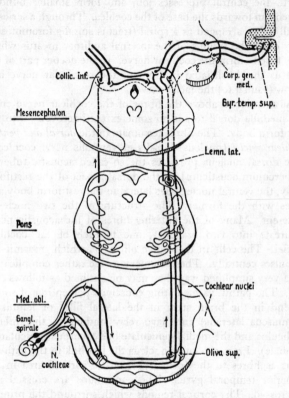

Fig. 11. A simplified diagram of the central auditory pathways.
(From Brodal, 1949.)

Most of the lemniscus fibres terminate in the inferior colliculus, but some appear to run directly to the medial geniculate body. Most of the afferents to the latter are, however, axons of cells in the inferior colliculus. Some of them cross the midline (Barnes, Magoun and Ranson, 1943). The large number of fibres from the inferior colliculus to the medial geniculate body constitute the inferior quadrigeminal brachium (brachium quadrigeminum inferius) which is visible to the naked eye. For an account of the termination of these fibres see Moore and Goldberg (1963).

The fibres from the dorsal cochlear nucleus are frequently stated to make up the macroscopically visible *medullary striae* (striae medullares) in the floor of the 4th ventricle. Recent investigations indicate, however, that these fibres in the acoustic system (which in man are scantier than those from the ventral nucleus) take a more profound course, and that the visible striae are formed by fibres which are related to the cerebellum and connect this with the pontobulbar body (Alphin and Barnes, 1944; Rasmussen and Peyton, 1946). Fibres from the cerebral cortex also end in the medial geniculate body and the inferior colliculus. These fibres, as well as the efferent olivo-cochlear bundle of Rasmussen (1953) appear to influence the central transmission of acoustic impulses (see Desmedt, 1960).

Some of the nuclei in the acoustic pathways, for example the superior olive (Rasmussen, 1946; Stotler, 1953), give off fibres to the reticular formation of the brain stem. Likewise the lateral lemniscus gives off collaterals to it. Such fibres form part of reflex arcs in various *acoustic reflexes*, by influencing, directly or via intercalated neurons, cells in the motor cranial nerve nuclei. The inferior colliculus appears to be an important acoustic reflex centre.

Just as in the optic system, *there exists within the acoustic system a distinct localization*: impulses arising from different parts of the organ of Corti in response to sounds of different frequencies are transmitted to particular discrete regions within the cortical acoustic area. Sounds of different frequency are thus 'represented' in this in an orderly sequence (tonotopic localization).

This localization has been established by anatomical and physiological investigations, and its presence also in man is supported by the results of clinico-pathological studies. In the cochlea high-pitched sounds are perceived in its basal turn, low-pitched sounds in the apical. Experimental research shows that this localization is very clear cut. The fibres from different parts of the cochlear spiral end in a localized manner in the cochlear nuclei (Lewy and Kobrak, 1936). By means of micro-electrode recordings this pattern has been mapped in great detail (Rose, Galambos and Hughes, 1959). Following small lesions in the cortical acoustic area, the ensuing retrograde cellular loss in the medial geniculate body is sharply localized (Walker and Fulton, 1938). So far it has not been possible by anatomical methods to define a corresponding localization in the projection from the cochlear nuclei to the inferior colliculus. However, a localization must be assumed to exist, since physiological studies unequivocally are in favour of it. In response to stimulation by sounds of different frequencies action potentials can be recorded in sharply delimited regions of the acoustic cortex in various animals, for example the chimpanzee (Bailey, von Bonin, Garol and McCulloch, 1943). This localization has been mapped out in detail particularly by Tunturi (1950).

Function and Clinical Aspects

The function of the cochlear nerve is examined by applying tests of hearing. In addition to simple tests, such as examining the patient's ability to hear a whispering voice, audiometry is now in ordinary use. This method permits an exact determination of the hearing capacity for sounds of different frequencies. A reduction of hearing can also be assessed quantitatively. A comparison between the bony conduction of sound (through the skull) and air conduction (through the tympanic cavity with the ossicles of the ear) permits an orientation as to whether a loss of hearing depends on a deficient conduction of sound (for example in an inflammation of the middle ear) or whether the receptor organ or the cochlear nerve is suffering. (In the former case the patient will perceive the sound of a vibrating tuning fork better when it is placed on the bony mastoid process than when it is held near the auricle.) Lesions of the cochlear nerve (or of the cochlea itself) will result in reduced hearing on the affected side. Pathological processes in the nerve (or in the cochlea), which produce irritation of the nerve fibres, will frequently result in subjective acoustic phenomena (tinnitus aurium). On account of the partial crossing of the central acoustic pathways, unilateral damage to them, or an affection of one acoustic cortical area, will not result in a definite reduction of hearing. However, subjectively perceived sounds may occur in such cases, occasionally as an initial symptom (aura) in an epileptic seizure.

The *cochlear nerve may be damaged* in fractures of the

temporal bone. Most frequently the nerve is affected by acoustic nerve tumours (p. 77). In the beginning tinnitus is frequent, in the later course a reduction of hearing becomes manifest. On account of their proximity to the cochlear nerve, the vestibular and facial nerves will frequently be involved simultaneously. In later stages symptoms may occur which are due to affection of the trigeminal nerve, particularly its first branch, and of the brain stem and the cerebellum. Inflammations on the base of the brain may involve the cochlear nerve. Disturbances in the function of hearing are, however, far more frequently due to diseases of the middle and inner ear than to affections of the cochlear nerve.

The Facial Nerve
(and the Intermediate Nerve)

Anatomy

The 7th cranial nerve, the facial, is the nerve which supplies the muscles of facial expression, and is *somatic efferent*. It runs together with the *intermediate nerve* (nervus intermedius), which may be considered as a *sensory root of the facial nerve* and in addition carries *visceral efferent fibres*. The facial is the nerve of the 2nd branchial arch.

The facial nerve emerges as a fairly large fibre bundle at the caudal border of the pons (figs. 5 and 8), in front of the statoacoustic nerve and the flocculus. This region is often called the *cerebellopontine* angle. The fibres of the intermediate nerve form a small bundle between the facial and the stato-acoustic nerves, and the intermediate joins these two nerves in their course to the fundus of the internal auditory meatus. Here the facial nerve is situated anteriorly (frontally) and superiorly (rostrally). The nerves are surrounded by a common dural sheath. From the fundus of the internal auditory meatus the facial and intermediate nerves continue in their own bony channel, the facial canal (canalis facialis). In its first part this is directed laterally, but at the so-called *facial knee*, the *geniculum of the facial nerve*, it makes a sharp bend in a posterior direction. At the genu the intermediate nerve shows a small swelling, the *geniculate ganglion* (ganglion geniculi, fig. 12) which contains the pseudounipolar perikarya of its afferent fibres. From the genu the canal with its nerves runs horizontally in a posterior (dorsal) direction. In this part of its course

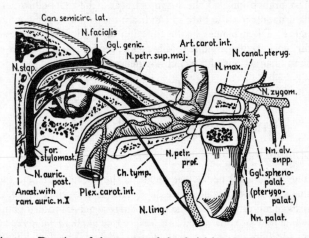

Fig. 12. Drawing of the course of the facial-intermediate nerve in the temporal bone.

it is found close to the wall of the tympanic cavity. Above the oval window (fenestra vestibuli) and below the lateral semicircular canal it produces an elongated bulging. The canal with the nerves then makes a second bend and its final course is directed downwards to the *stylomastoid foramen*, where the facial nerve leaves the skull. Shortly before it reaches the foramen, the facial nerve has an anastomosis with the auricular ramus of the vagus nerve. (The majority of the fibres of the intermediate nerve leave the canal more proximally, see below.)

In the first part of its *extracranial course* the facial nerve is embedded in the parotid gland and runs in a posteroinferiorly convex arch lateral to the external carotid artery to the lateral aspect of the cheek. In the parotid gland, a *plexus* (plexus parotidicus) is formed, from which the terminal branches of the nerve emerge (fig. 16). An anastomosis between the plexus and the auriculotemporal nerve (from the mandibular nerve) enables the secretory fibres from the otic ganglion to reach the parotid gland (see p. 87). Before the facial nerve splits into its terminal branches, it gives off a *posterior auricular branch* (ramus auricularis posterior) which ascends behind the auricle and supplies the extrinsic muscles of the ear and the occipital muscle. Another branch innervates the posterior belly of the digrastric muscle and the stylohyoid muscle. Furthermore, the nerve has an anastomosis with the glossopharyngeal nerve at the petrosal ganglion (belonging to the latter nerve).

The upper *terminal branches of the facial nerve* run from the parotid plexus anteriorly across the zygomatic arch to the frontal, orbicularis oculi and corrugator supercilii muscles. Other branches course horizontally to the zygomatic, orbicularis oris and other muscles surrounding the mouth, including the buccinator muscle. A caudal branch, the *ramus colli*, runs in an anterior direction below the lower jaw and supplies the platysma (anastomoses with cutaneous branches from the cervical plexus). The branches which have been enumerated all carry somatic efferent fibres to the striated mimetic musculature which is developed from the mesenchyme of the 2nd branchial arch.

The *fibres of the intermediate nerve* and a few fibres of the facial nerve leave the nerves during their course in the facial canal as three branches (fig. 12). Some somatic efferent facial nerve fibres take off as the *stapedial nerve* (nervus stapedius) at the place where the canal runs in the posterior wall of the tympanic cavity and innervates the stapedius muscle. The *greater superficial petrosal nerve* (nervus petrosus superficialis major) leaves the intermediate nerve at the geniculate ganglion, and through a small opening, the hiatus of the facial canal, it enters the cranial cavity. It runs forward on the surface of the pyramid of the temporal bone and passes below

67

the semilunar ganglion and lateral to the internal carotid artery through the foramen lacerum. It then joins the *deep petrosal nerve* (nervus petrosus profundus) from the sympathetic plexus around the internal carotid, to form the *nerve of the pterygoid canal* (nervus canalis pterygoidei, Vidian nerve).

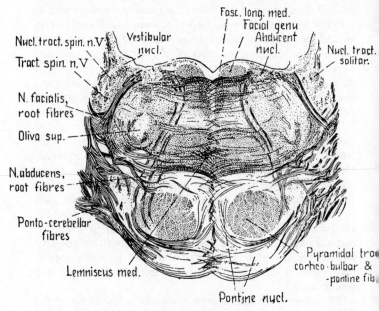

Fig. 13. Drawing of a myelin-stained transverse section through the pons. (From Brodal, 1949.)

Through the pterygoid canal this nerve passes to the spheno-palatine fossa and ends in the sphenopalatine ganglion. In this way visceral efferent fibres from the intermediate nerve reach the sphenopalatine ganglion (fig. 17). Postganglionic fibres from this then mediate secretory impulses to the lacrimal gland (via the zygomatic nerve and its anastomosis with the lacrimal nerve). Other postganglionic fibres from the ganglion carry secretory impulses to glands in the nasal cavity. Taste fibres from the soft palate run centrally in the greater superficial petrosal nerve (fig. 14).

The other branch from the intermediate nerve, the *chorda tympani*, leaves the nerve in the facial canal just below the stapedial nerve (fig. 12). It enters the tympanic cavity through a small bony canal, courses anteriorly in a rostrally convex arch in the cavity (covered by the mucous membrane) and leaves it through the petrotympanic fissure. It then runs ventrocaudally to the posterior aspect of the lingual nerve with which it fuses. In this way secretory (preganglionic parasympathetic) fibres to the submandibular and sublingual gland and the small glands in the oral cavity are brought into the lingual nerve (see p. 84 and fig. 17). The visceral afferent taste fibres from the anterior two-thirds of the tongue run in a central direction via the lingual nerve and the chorda tympani. These fibres have their perikarya in the geniculate ganglion (see p. 66 and fig. 14).

The *motor, somatic efferent fibres of the facial nerve* are axons from the cells of the *motor facial nucleus* which belongs to the special somatic efferent nuclei (fig. 3). The nucleus forms a distinct collection of large multipolar cells in the caudal part of the pons, rostral to the nucleus ambiguus. Immediately rostral to the nucleus is the superior olive (fig. 13). In early foetal life the facial nucleus is developed just underneath the floor of the 4th ventricle, but later it migrates in a ventral direction. The first part of the fibres of the facial nerve, therefore, ultimately come to have an arched course in the brain stem. When traced from the nucleus, they first run in a dorsomedial direction and then turn rostrally in a sharp bend dorsal to the nucleus of the abducent nerve. (In this way a small elevation, the facial colliculus, is produced in the floor of 4th ventricle.) From the bend, the *facial genu* (genu nervi facialis), the fibres finally run ventrolaterally (fig. 13) and emerge at the lower border of the pons (fig. 5).

Corticobulbar fibres, which course together with the pyramidal tract, are assumed to mediate impulses initiating voluntary movements of the facial muscles (see p. 24). In addition the *facial nucleus may be activated* by impulses from subcortical regions (particularly the globus pallidus and hypothalamus), which presumably play a role in the emotional innervation of the mimetic muscles (see below). Furthermore, afferent impulses entering in various cranial nerves may elicit reflexes in which the efferent link of the reflex arc is formed by fibres of the facial nerve (for example the blink reflex: closure of the eyelids on touching the cornea; reflex contraction of the stapedius muscle on loud noises, and so-called acoustico-facial reflexes: contractions of mimetic muscles on unexpected loud sounds). However, none of the fibres which can activate the cells of the facial nucleus appear to end directly on its cells.

The cells of the facial nucleus are arranged in incompletely separated groups. Experimental studies indicate that different muscles are supplied by particular cell groups. The fibres coursing in the upper branches of the facial nerve are derived from the ventral parts of the nucleus, the fibres of the lower branches from its dorsal parts (Szentágothai, 1948b). It is of interest that the muscles above the palpebral fissure are supplied from a well-defined portion of the nucleus (Vraa-Jensen, 1942), since this part of the nucleus appears to be influenced by crossed as well as uncrossed corticobulbar fibres, while the rest of the nucleus is controlled by the contralateral cortex only. This is of relevance in the differential diagnosis between central and peripheral facial palsies (see below).

In man the facial nerve contains some 7000 fibres. Three-quarters of these are myelinated and most of them are relatively thick, 7-10 μ (van Buskirk, 1945). Probably fibres from one nucleus pass only to homolateral muscles. The motor units in the mimetic muscles must be assumed to be relatively small, particularly in man, whose almost infinitely varying facial expressions depend on a finely differentiated innervation of the many mimetic muscles. In man the units in the platysma have been determined to consist of about 25 muscle fibres (Feinstein and others, 1954).

The *visceral efferent fibres of the intermediate nerve* are assumed to come from a small *superior salivatory nucleus*[1] (nucleus salivatorius superior s. pontis) situated rostral to

[1] According to the recent study of Torvik (1957a) the superior and inferior salivatory nuclei are diffuse aggregations of cells, which fuse into each other.

the dorsal motor vagus nucleus (fig. 3). As described above these preganglionic parasympathetic fibres pass in part in the greater superficial petrosal nerve to the sphenopalatine ganglion, in part in the chorda tympani and the lingual nerve to the submandibular ganglion.[1] Secretion of saliva and tears on

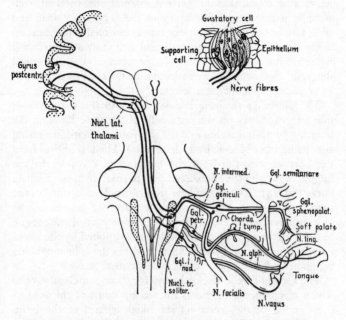

Fig. 14. Diagram of the pathways for taste. (From Brodal, 1949.)

reflex or psychic stimuli is initiated by fibres which (presumably by way of intercalated neurons) activate the cells of the salivatory nucleus.

The *visceral afferent fibres of the intermediate nerve* which have their perikarya in the geniculate ganglion terminate in the

[1] In the cat and dog some 70 per cent of all visceral efferent fibres of the intermediate nerve pass in the greater superficial petrosal nerve, only some 30 per cent in the chorda tympani (Foley and DuBois, 1943).

71

rostral part of the nucleus of the solitary tract (fig. 14). Most of these fibres run centrally in the greater superficial petrosal nerve and the chorda tympani. They transmit impulses of taste and would thus be classified as special visceral afferent. However, there are reasons to assume that the intermediate nerve also contains some general visceral afferent and even some somatic afferent fibres. Since the nerves are small and their number of fibres of various types restricted, a clarification of the details meets with great difficulties. Only a few relevant data will be mentioned, but, on account of their practical diagnostic importance, the pathways for the taste impulses will be considered somewhat more closely.

The *pathways for taste impulses* begin in the periphery as fine afferent fibres on the taste cells of the taste buds on the tongue, the palatal arches and the soft palate. (With increasing age the number of taste buds decreases.) The taste fibres from the anterior two-thirds of the tongue run centrally in the lingual nerve and the chorda tympani to reach the intermediate nerve (fig. 14). The taste fibres from the posterior third of the tongue, including the large vallate papillae, course in the glossopharyngeal nerve. A small posterior part of the tongue and the upper surface of the epiglottis is supplied by the vagus nerve. From the soft palate fibres pass via the sphenopalatine ganglion and the greater superficial petrosal nerve.[1]

The second link in the pathways for those impulses of taste which reach consciousness is formed by axons of the cells of the nucleus of the solitary tract which ascend in the brain stem (fig. 14). These pathways may be followed to the 'face region' in the lateral thalamic nucleus (nucleus ventralis posteromedialis thalami). They appear to run with the medial lemniscus in close relation to ascending secondary trigeminal

[1] In some cases surgical section of the chorda tympani has not been followed by loss of the sense of taste in the anterior two-thirds of the tongue (Schwarz and Weddell, 1938), and it has been assumed that the taste fibres in these cases, after having followed the distal part of the chorda tympani, enter the greater superficial petrosal nerve via anastomoses with the otic ganglion. Such conditions may result in diagnostic errors in the determination of the seat of an injury to the facial nerve (see below and Brodal, 1948).

fibres (Gerebtzoff, 1939). Bilateral destruction of this nucleus in monkeys results in loss of the sense of taste (Patton, Ruch and Walker, 1944). In agreement with the projection of this nucleus on the 'face region' in the cortical sensory area in the posterior central gyrus, it emerges from experimental studies and from clinical observations in man (Börnstein, 1940; Penfield and Erickson, 1941) that the cortical 'taste area' must be situated here. In unilateral affections of this region the sense of taste may be abolished on the contralateral half of the tongue. In addition to the fibres to the thalamus, the nucleus of the solitary tract sends fibres to the hypothalamus, and collaterals or axons may also transmit impulses to efferent cranial nerve nuclei, particularly the visceral efferent ones, as links in reflex arcs (for example for secretion of saliva).

Even if most of the afferent fibres of the intermediate nerve are visceral, there are also some *somatic afferent fibres*. They can be traced to the nucleus of the spinal trigeminal tract (Pearson, 1945, and others). Some of them pass via anastomoses with the auricular ramus of the vagus nerve to the skin in the concha of the auricle. Others appear to run peripherally with the fibres of the facial nerve. It might be conjectured that they are *proprioceptive* fibres from the mimetic muscles, which must be assumed to be amply supplied with proprioceptive receptors.

Experimental studies (Foley and DuBois, 1943) make it likely, however, that only few sensory fibres are found in the facial nerve distal to the stylomastoid foramen. According to Bruesch (1944) only 8 per cent of the afferent fibres pass in the muscular branches. Most of these fibres are thin, 1·5-6 μ, and are, therefore, assumed to be pain fibres. Ordinary muscle spindles have not so far been described in the mimetic muscles, except for the platysma (Feinstein and others, 1954). It is conceivable that the proprioceptive receptors may be of another type in these muscles than in the common skeletal muscles. The fact that some fibres of the intermediate nerve can be traced to the mesencephalic trigeminal nucleus (Pearson, 1945) lends some support to the contention that the afferent fibres in the facial nerve may mediate proprioceptive impulses, since this nucleus appears to be related to proprioceptive impulses from the masticatory muscles and the extrinsic eye muscles. It appears unlikely, however, that the

73

few afferent fibres in the facial nerve may be sufficient to subserve proprioception from the mimetic muscles. Some clinical observations (following interruptions of the trigeminal nerve and other lesions) have been interpreted as demonstrating a central conduction of such proprioceptive impulses in the trigeminal nerve, but yet other clinical experiences have been taken to exclude this possibility. The question of the proprioceptive innervation of the mimetic muscles is thus still open.

Function

The *chief function of the facial-intermediate nerve* is to mediate impulses to movements of the muscles of facial expression. Its role in the pathways for taste, in the innervation of the lacrimal and salivary glands and of the skin in the concha of the auricle is of less importance. The *motor function* of the nerve is examined by testing the movements of the mimetic muscles in acts such as closing the eyelids, frowning, blowing out a candle (buccinator muscle), showing the teeth, whistling, etc. The power on contraction may also be tested. On inspection an asymmetry between the two halves of the face can be observed, likewise atrophy, contracture, fascicular twitchings (see p. 27) and involuntary movements. The *sense of taste* is tested by applying particles of substances of different taste (salt, sugar, quinine, citric acid) on the tongue. The patient may have observed alterations in the *secretory functions* (of tears or saliva). These functions may be tested by eliciting reflex secretions from the lacrimal and salivary glands.

Clinical Aspects

Affections of the facial-intermediate nerve may be followed by disturbances in any of its functional spheres. The site of the lesion will determine the symptoms which will appear in the individual case. This follows from the anatomical features, and an analysis of the symptoms, therefore, frequently makes possible a topical diagnosis of the lesion. The motor symptoms are the most important ones and will be considered first.

Facial palsy is the most commonly occurring of the cranial

74

nerve paralyses. Most frequent is an affection of the nerve itself, an infranuclear paralysis (see p. 26 and fig. 4). If some of the branches only are involved, for example in diseases of the parotid gland or wounds in this region, the paralysis will be restricted to some only of the facial muscles. Far more commonly the entire nerve is affected. As a rule there will then be widespread loss of motor function, but this may not be complete. If all facial nerve fibres are *completely interrupted*, the mimetic muscles on the affected side will *loose their tonus* and gradually become *atrophic*. The normal wrinkles and creases in the face, due to the insertion of muscle fibres in the skin, will become less marked. The affected side of the face acquires a smooth, empty expression. The angle of the mouth on this side will be drooping. The patient is unable to draw the angle of the mouth laterally (when trying to show his teeth), the eye cannot be closed. (Concerning the so-called Bell's palsy see p. 78.) The patient cannot frown, is unable to whistle, his speech suffers (particularly the labial consonants). Reflex contractions are abolished (for example the corneal reflex). On account of the paralysis of the orbicularis oculi muscle the cornea is in danger of drying with resultant formation of corneal ulcer. In a *paresis* the symptoms will be less marked, and the power on contraction of the muscles on the two sides should be compared.[1]

The same symptoms will appear in *nuclear facial palsy*, where the facial nucleus is affected. Fascicular twitching may be seen in such instances. On account of the localization within the facial nucleus (see p. 70) occasionally the paralysis or paresis may be limited to certain muscle groups only.

A *supranuclear facial palsy* is seen in lesions of the corticobulbar fibres from the face subdivision of the motor cortex

---

[1] In many cases of peripheral facial palsies after some time a contracture of the muscles on the paretic side appears, revealing itself most clearly by the angle of the mouth being drawn laterally. At first sight it may appear as if the paretic side is the normal one. The reasons for the appearance of a facial contracture are obscure. According to Taverner (1955) the contracture is due to steady, low-frequency activity of some motor units.

which supply the facial nucleus (see p. 69), for example as part of a hemiplegia following a cerebral apoplexy, or in lesions of the cortex itself. Since the part of the facial nucleus which innervates the muscles above the palpebral fissure, is supplied from both cerebral hemispheres (see p. 70) a central facial paralysis of this type will affect only the muscles below the palpebral fissure on the contralateral side. The patient is thus able to close his eye and frown on the paretic side of the face. Furthermore, there will be no atrophy and the facial reflexes are preserved. In doubtful cases electromyography may be of diagnostic value (Weddell, Feinstein and Pattle, 1944).

A peculiar phenomenon which occurs in central facial palsy of this type is a *dissociation between the voluntary and the emotional facial innervation.* In spite of the patient's inability to show his teeth when asked to do so, he will smile spontaneously when he enjoys a joke.

It may then even be observed that the smile, as well as other emotional mimetic expressions, starts earlier and lasts longer on the paretic side of the face than on the other (Monrad-Krohn, 1924). It may be assumed that descending fibres from higher levels other than the cerebral cortex (? basal ganglia, ? hypothalamus) mediate the impulses to the emotional facial movements, while in the voluntary, 'social', smile presumably the corticobulbar fibres are engaged. In agreement with this explanation, reduced expression (poker face) is seen in lesions of the basal ganglia, for example in paralysis agitans. In Huntington's chorea involuntary movements in the face are a frequent initial symptom.

Loss of taste in the anterior two-thirds of the tongue in facial palsy points to an interruption of the visceral afferent fibres of the homolateral intermediate nerve. On account of the course of this nerve, a loss of taste in this distribution may occur in combination with loss of facial motor function in any lesion which involves these nerves between their exit from the pons (and within the pons) and the departure of the chorda tympani.[1]

[1] As mentioned above, in some individuals the taste fibres in the intermediate nerve appear not to run in the chorda tympani. In this case, loss of taste will occur only in lesions central to the geniculate ganglion. This possibility should be kept in mind in diagnostic considerations of the possible site of a facial nerve lesion.

Loss of taste without motor symptoms will occur if the chorda tympani is affected in the tympanic cavity or further peripherally in its course, and may also follow lesions of the lingual nerve (in the latter case the anaesthesia of the tongue will be a diagnostic clue).

Disturbances in the *secretion of saliva* will occur in the same lesions which produce loss of taste, since the secretory fibres follow the same route as the taste fibres. The *secretion of tears*, however, will suffer only in lesions situated central to the geniculate ganglion (since the visceral efferent fibres to the lacrimal gland run in the greater superficial petrosal nerve). The so-called 'syndrome of crocodile tears' is described on p. 125. A final symptom of some focal diagnostic value is the so-called *hyperacusis* (acoustic sensations are increased on the affected side). This phenomenon appears to be due to a paralysis of the stapedius muscle. This symptom will only be seen if the facial nerve is affected central to the departure of the nerve to the stapedius.[1]

There are many possible *causes for peripheral infranuclear facial palsies*. In the cerebellopontine angle or in the first part of the internal auditory meatus the facial nerve will usually be involved at an early stage when a so-called acoustic nerve tumour develops (neurinomas arising from the Schwann cells in the nerve sheaths). As a rule there are at the same time symptoms from the stato-acoustic nerve (see pp. 60 and 65) and cerebellar symptoms. During its course in the facial canal, the nerve is particularly exposed where the canal runs close to the tympanic cavity (otitis, mastoiditis). Skull fractures through the temporal bone may cause a facial palsy. Tumours of the parotid gland, open wounds and surgical incisions carried across the direction of the fibres may affect the nerve extracranially. In leprosy partial facial palsies are common. In most cases of peripheral facial palsies, however, no definite

[1] A reduction of the cutaneous sensibility in the concha of the auricle can scarcely be detected in a lesion of the intermediate nerve, since the vagus and glossopharyngeal nerves take part in the innervation of this region.

cause can be ascertained. It is common then to speak of a 'rheumatic facial palsy' (Bell's palsy) because the symptoms frequently start in relation to an infection, an 'influenza' or following exposure to a draught.

It has been assumed that the cause for this type of facial palsy (which commonly recedes completely after some time) is oedema in the facial canal, leading to a compression of the nerve with an ensuing abolition of the power of conduction in the nerve fibres. Surgical opening of the canal and decompression of the nerve have been reported to give good results in many cases, but pathological proof that the current conception of the cause of the palsy is correct, has not been brought forward. Anatomical studies make it clear that there must be ample room for the nerve in the canal, since the nerve nowhere occupies more than 50 per cent of the entire cross-sectional area of the canal, the rest being filled by connective tissue and vessels (Sunderland and Cossar, 1953). Taverner (1955) brings forward good arguments against operation in cases of ordinary 'rheumatic' facial palsies.

Nuclear facial palsy, due to an affection of the cells of the facial nucleus, may be seen in poliomyelitis and progressive bulbar paralysis. In addition to the symptoms seen following an interruption of the facial nerve (infranuclear palsy), fascicular twitchings may occur, while symptoms from the intermediate nerve will be lacking. Also in tumours, inflammations and vascular lesions in the pons facial palsy may occur when the lesion affects the facial nucleus or the root fibres of the nerve in their course in the pons. As a rule other structures will then be involved simultaneously, for example the abducent nucleus or the pyramidal tract. In rare cases a congenital facial palsy is met with, depending on defective development of the facial nucleus.

Supranuclear facial palsies are most commonly seen in conjunction with capsular hemiplegia, and are then found on the side contralateral to the lesion. In pseudobulbar palsy, the paresis is usually bilateral and combined with symptoms from other motor cranial nerves.

Isolated *symptoms from the intermediate nerve* are seen in so-called *geniculate neuralgia*. Pains localized to the external ear and the external auditory meatus, sometimes also deep in the face (fibres in the greater superficial petrosal nerve), occur in paroxysms. Sometimes pain is also felt in the areas of the glossopharyngeal and trigeminal nerves ('irradiation'). Before or contemporaneously with the pain, vesicles may appear in the external auditory meatus or on the auricle, so-called *otic herpes* (occasionally also on the soft palate). This is assumed to be due to an inflammation of the geniculate ganglion. Facial palsy may accompany it.[1]

The Trigeminal Nerve

Anatomy

The 5th cranial nerve, the trigeminal, is the nerve of the 1st branchial arch. It supplies the face and its cavities with *general somatic afferent fibres* and carries *special somatic efferent fibres* to the masticatory muscles. The nerve is the largest of the cranial nerves.

The trigeminal nerve leaves the brain stem about half way between the lower and upper borders of the pons on its ventrolateral aspect (fig. 5). Even with the naked eye it is seen that the fibres form two bundles, a larger lateral *portio major*, and a much smaller, medial *portio minor*. The former is the sensory, the latter the motor root (fig. 8).

The nerve takes a ventral and slightly ascending course through the pontine cistern and pierces the dura mater just below the attachment of the tentorium cerebelli (fig. 15). About 1 cm. from the pons the larger portio major swells to the large *Gasserian or semilunar ganglion* (ganglion semilunare) composed of pseudounipolar nerve cells. The ganglion is flattened and rests in a small groove (impressio trigemini) on

[1] Geniculate neuralgia has been cured in some cases by surgical section of the intermediate nerve central to the ganglion. Since the pain fibres in the intermediate nerve pass to the spinal trigeminal nucleus, it is possible that a medullary tractotomy (Sjöqvist operation) may be of therapeutic value.

the temporal pyramid near its apex. It is here enclosed in a 'pouch' of the dura with a lower and an upper wall. Below the ganglion the greater and lesser superficial petrosal nerves run ventrally, medial to it is the cavernous sinus with the internal carotid artery. From the ganglion the *three chief divisions of the trigeminal nerve* take off. These are: the *1st division, the ophthalmic nerve; the 2nd division, the maxillary nerve, and the 3rd division, the mandibular nerve*. The portio minor runs below the ganglion and joins the mandibular nerve. Therefore,

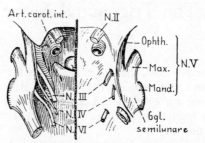

Fig. 15. The relations of the cranial nerves in the cavernous sinus. The dura has been removed on the left side.

all motor fibres of the trigeminal nerve are distributed with this division. The three principal divisions give off numerous smaller branches.

1. The *ophthalmic nerve* (nervus ophthalmicus) passes in a ventral and slightly rostral direction through the cavernous sinus, where it receives some fibres from the sympathetic plexus on the internal carotid artery. In the sinus the nerve is found below the trochlear nerve, lateral to the abducent and oculomotor nerves (fig. 15). It gives off a small *tentorial ramus* (ramus tentorii) which supplies part of the dura mater, and continues through the superior orbital fissure to the orbit, where it subdivides into three terminal branches: the lacrimal, the frontal and the nasociliary nerves.

The *lacrimal nerve* (nervus lacrimalis) is the most lateral of these, running underneath the roof of the orbit to the lacrimal gland. By an anastomosis with the zygomatic nerve it receives postganglionic secretory fibres to the gland. These fibres have their perikarya in the sphenopalatine ganglion. The nerve

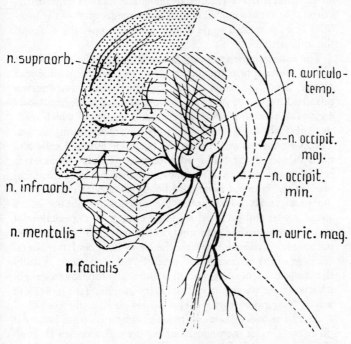

Fig. 16. The distribution of the chief cutaneous branches of the trigeminal nerve. Stippled: area of the ophthalmic division. Horizontal hatchings: area of the maxillary division. Oblique hatchings: area of the mandibular division. (Redrawn after Corning.)

also carries afferent fibres from the lacrimal gland and its surroundings.

The *frontal nerve* (nervus frontalis) is the largest of the three branches. It runs ventrally underneath the roof of the orbit (above the levator palpebrae muscle) and splits into several

81

branches. The largest of these is the *supraorbital nerve* (nervus supraorbitalis) which emerges on the forehead through the supraorbital foramen (or incisure) and supplies the skin of the forehead as far up as the vertex (fig. 16). The minor branches of the frontal nerve (ramus frontalis and nervus supratrochlearis) take a more medial course to the medial part of the forehead and the medial angle of the eye and supply the skin and the conjunctiva.

The *nasociliary nerve* (nervus nasociliaris) is the medialmost branch of the ophthalmic nerve. It approaches the medial wall of the orbit, and ends as the infratrochlear nerve (nervus infratrochlearis). It gives off the *anterior and posterior ethmoid nerves* (nervus ethmoideus anterior and posterior) which leave the orbit through small holes with corresponding names. The posterior nerve supplies the posterior ethmoid cells and the sphenoid sinus. The anterior nerve enters the anterior cranial fossa, courses for a short distance on the cribriform plate of the ethmoid bone, and finally penetrates this to enter the nasal cavity. It supplies the mucous membrane in its anterior part and gives off a special branch, the *external nasal ramus* (ramus nasalis externus), to the nose. This branch becomes subcutaneous between the nasal bone and the lateral cartilage of the nose and innervates the tip of the nose. Finally the nasociliary nerve gives off a branch (radix longa ganglii ciliaris) to the parasympathetic ciliary ganglion (see p. 85) and sensory *long ciliary nerves* (nervi ciliares longi) to the eyeball.

2. The *maxillary nerve*. From the cavernous sinus (where it gives off a small meningeal ramus) the nerve passes through the foramen rotundum in the pterygoid bone to the sphenopalatine fossa (fig. 12). The bulk of the fibres continue as the large *infraorbital nerve* (nervus infraorbitalis) which runs in a ventral direction in the floor of the orbit, first in the infraorbital sulcus, then in the infraorbital canal. It emerges through the infraorbital foramen and splits into several branches which supply the skin on the surface of the maxilla down as far as the mouth (fig. 16) and on the lower eyelid (rami nasales, labiales and palpebrales inferiores, respectively).

A relatively large branch from the maxillary (or infraorbital) nerve is the *zygomatic nerve* (nervus zygomaticus). It runs along the lateral wall of the orbit and gives off small branches which penetrate the zygomatic bone and supply the skin covering this and the anterior part of the temple (ramus zygomaticofacialis and ramus zygomaticotemporalis). The zygomatic nerve, as mentioned previously, has an anastomosis with the lacrimal nerve.

Several *superior dental nerves* (nervi alveolares superiores) take off from the infraorbital nerve. They supply the teeth in the upper jaw (fig. 12). The most posterior branches (nervi alveolares superiores posteriores) first course superficially on the surface of the maxillary tuberosity before they enter small bony channels and supply the molar teeth. A middle branch (nervus alveolaris superior medius) runs in an individual channel to the premolars, and the anterior branches (nervi alveolares superiores anteriores) pass in fine channels in the anterior wall of the maxillary sinus to the canine and incisor teeth. The fibres form a *dental plexus* (plexus dentalis superior) above the alveoli of the teeth and innervate these and the surrounding gums. Many of these branches run in small furrows in the wall of the maxillary sinus in intimate contact with its mucous membrane. This is of some practical importance.

The last branches of the maxillary nerve are the *sphenopalatine nerves* (nervi sphenopalatini). These take a descending course, some of them enter the sphenopalatine ganglion, but most of them bypass it. Some minor branches (rami orbitales) pass to the posteromedial part of the orbit, others enter the nasal cavity (rami nasales posteriores) through the sphenopalatine foramen and supply the mucous membrane in the posterior part of the nasal cavity. One of the branches, called the *long sphenopalatine nerve* (nervus nasopalatinus), runs in an anterior and descending direction on the nasal septum and through the incisive canal it pierces the hard palate. The larger posterior part of the latter and the soft palate are supplied by the greater and lesser *palatine nerves* (nervi palatini, fig. 12). These descend from the sphenopalatine fossa in the canales palatini to the palate and spread in the anterior (nervus palatinus major), medial (nervus palatinus medius) and posterior (nervus palatinus minor) direction.

3. The *mandibular nerve*. This carries all the motor fibres of the trigeminal nerve, and is the largest of the three principal trigeminal divisions. It leaves the skull through the oval foramen. (It gives off a recurrent branch, the nervus spinosus, through the foramen spinosum to the dura.) The mandibular nerve splits into several branches. The *masticatory nerve* (nervus masticatorius) is the name of a group of short branches which chiefly carry motor fibres to the four masticatory muscles: the temporal, masseter, external and internal pterygoid, as well as to the tensor veli palati and tensor tympani muscles.

The *auriculotemporal nerve* (nervus auriculotemporalis) is a purely sensory branch which bends laterally, bifurcates around the middle meningeal artery and unites again to pass posterior to the neck of the mandible and enter the parotid gland. Within this it anastomoses with branches of the facial nerve, ascends superficial to the zygomatic arch together with the superficial temporal artery and supplies the skin of the temple and the anterior upper part of the auricle (fig. 16). The nerve has a connexion with the otic ganglion. In this way the postganglionic secretory fibres from this ganglion to the parotid gland reach the parotid plexus.

The *lingual nerve* (nervus lingualis) takes a ventral and descending course between the external and internal pterygoid muscles to the base of the tongue. It enters the latter between the hyoglossus and mylohyoid muscles and supplies the mucous membrane of the anterior two-thirds of the tongue with general somatic sensory fibres. During its arched course the lingual nerve receives the chorda tympani (figs. 12 and 14). This brings taste fibres and (parasympathetic) visceral efferent fibres into the nerve, but most of the latter leave it again to end in the submandibular ganglion (see below).

The *long buccal nerve* (nervus buccinatorius) is a smaller branch which passes between the internal and external pterygoid muscles (or through the latter) to the outer surface of the

84

buccinator muscle. It splits into many branches which penetrate the muscle and supply the mucous membrane on the inside of the cheek. Smaller branches supply the skin of the cheek. The nerve is purely sensory. (The buccinator muscle is innervated by the facial nerve.)

The *inferior dental nerve* (nervus alveolaris inferior s. mandibularis) is the largest branch of the mandibular nerve. Like the lingual nerve it takes an arched course in an anterior and inferior direction, a little lateral to, and below it, and enters the mandibular canal through the mandibular foramen. Before it enters the canal it gives off the *mylohyoid nerve* (nervus mylohyoideus) which runs along the under surface of the mylohyoid muscle, and innervates this and the anterior belly of the digastric muscle. In the canal the inferior dental nerve gives off numerous branches (rami dentales) to the alveoli and teeth, and as in the upper jaw these branches form a *dental plexus* (plexus dentalis inferior). The terminal branch of the nerve, the *mental nerve* (nervus mentalis, fig. 16) emerges from the mental foramen and supplies the skin of the lower lip and the chin.

In connexion with the description of the branches of the trigeminal nerve it will be appropriate to give a condensed account of the *parasympathetic ganglia which are related to the trigeminal divisions*. They are all collections of postganglionic, parasympathetic, neurons. The visceral efferent pathways are thus interrupted synaptically in these ganglia. However, the ganglia also contain fibres which pass through them. Some of these are sensory fibres (visceral or somatic afferent), others are visceral efferent, sympathetic, fibres. It has been customary to call the different groups of fibres 'roots' of the ganglia, and to distinguish a *motor root* (parasympathetic, radix motorica), a *sensory root* (radix sensitiva) and a *sympathetic root* (radix sympathica). Fig. 17 shows some principal features which will be described.

The *ciliary ganglion* (ganglion ciliare) which is related to the 1st trigeminal division, is found in the orbit as a flattened body lateral to the optic nerve (fig. 19). The *parasympathetic inflow* is represented

85

by visceral efferent fibres from the Edinger-Westphal nucleus which enter the ganglion as branches from the oculomotor nerve. The postganglionic fibres enter the eyeballs as 6-12 short ciliary nerves (nervi ciliares breves) and supply the ciliary muscle (accommodation) and the pupillary sphincter (constriction of the pupil). Together with these run (somatic) *sensory fibres* from the eyeball. They leave the

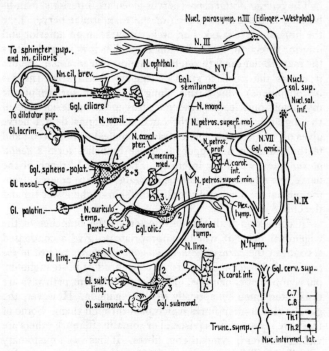

Fig. 17. Diagram of the parasympathetic ganglia in the head, and their fibre connexions. (From Jansen, 1955.)

ciliary ganglion in its sensory root: connexions with the nasociliary nerve (see p. 82). The *sympathetic root* is formed by fibres derived from the sympathetic plexus on the ophthalmic artery (postganglionic fibres, perikarya in the superior cervical ganglion of the sympathetic trunk). The sympathetic fibres reach the eyeball in the same way as the other fibres and are vasomotor.

The *sphenopalatine ganglion* (ganglion sphenopalatinum) belongs to the 2nd trigeminal division, the maxillary nerve, and is situated in the pterygopalatine fossa (fig. 12). Its *sensory root* is formed by con- nexions with the maxillary nerve via somatic afferent fibres from the nasal cavity and the palate which pass the ganglion (see p. 83). The *parasympathetic* and the majority of the *sympathetic fibres* to the ganglion enter it in the nerve of the pterygoid canal (nervus canalis pterygoidei), formed by the fusion of the greater superficial petrosal nerve and the deep petrosal nerve. The former (p. 67) carries preganglionic fibres from the superior salivatory nucleus, which establish synaptical contact with the perikarya of postganglionic neurons in the ganglion. By the connexions with the maxillary nerve secretory fibres find their way to the lacrimal gland and to glands in the posterior part of the nasal cavity (p. 68). The deep petrosal nerve is formed by postganglionic fibres of the sympathetic plexus around the internal carotid artery. They have their perikarya in the superior cervical ganglion of the sympathetic trunk.

The *submandibular ganglion* (ganglion submandibulare) which is related to the 3rd trigeminal division, the mandibular nerve, is found as a small body below the lingual nerve on the hyoglossus muscle, above the submandibular gland. The *sensory root* of the ganglion is represented by fibres which connect it with the lingual nerve. *Sympa- thetic fibres* come from the plexus surrounding the facial artery (external maxillary artery) which runs on the inner surface of the submandibular gland. These fibres are postganglionic and like the sensory ones pass through the ganglion. The *parasympathetic root* is made up of postganglionic visceral efferent fibres of the inter- mediate nerve. By way of the chorda tympani (p. 69) they enter the lingual nerve and from this pass to the ganglion (perikarya in the superior salivatory nucleus). Some of the postganglionic neurons in the submandibular ganglion send their axons back to the lingual nerve. Via its branches they reach the sublingual gland and the smaller glands in the area of distribution of the lingual nerve. Other postganglionic secretory fibres enter the submandibular gland.

The *otic ganglion* (ganglion oticum) forms a small node just outside the oval foramen, medial to the mandibular nerve which leaves the skull in the foramen. The *sensory root* of the ganglion is formed by fine fibres from the mandibular nerve. These pass through the ganglion and continue in the auriculotemporal nerve and other branches. The *sympathetic root* is represented by fibres from the plexus around the middle meningeal artery. *The parasympathetic root* is formed by the lesser superficial petrosal nerve (p. 52). The peri- karya of the fibres are in the inferior salivatory nucleus. The post- ganglionic, parasympathetic fibres from the otic ganglion enter the auriculotemporal nerve, and by anastomoses between this and the parotid plexus the parotid gland receives its secretory fibres.

The *nuclei which are related to the trigeminal nerve are two*: a somatic efferent, motor, nucleus and a highly differentiated somatic afferent nucleus. The *motor trigeminal nucleus* is the most rostral of the special somatic efferent nuclei (fig. 3). It is made up of large multipolar cells and is situated at the middle level of the pons, just medial to the principal sensory nucleus

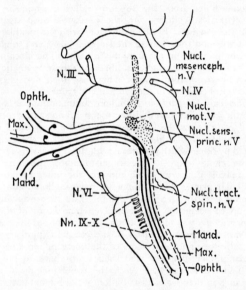

Fig. 18. Diagram of the differential distribution of the fibres of the three principal trigeminal divisions within the lower part of the nucleus of the spinal trigeminal tract. See text for explanation.

(see below), and immediately rostral to the motor facial nucleus. Its efferent fibres take a ventral course between the motor and principal sensory nucleus and emerge from the brain stem as the portio minor. As in the other motor cranial nerve nuclei, the various muscles supplied by the motor trigeminal nucleus receive their fibres from particular regions of it (Szentágothai, 1949).

The motor trigeminal nucleus is *acted upon by fibres from higher levels*, among them corticobulbar fibres (see p. 24 ff.). By way of intercalated cells sensory fibres from various cranial nerves may activate the nucleus in different reflex actions. Fibres from the mesencephalic trigeminal nucleus, however, end in direct synaptical contact with the cells of the motor nucleus (see below).

The *sensory trigeminal nucleus* forms a complex of nuclei which extends through the brain stem from the caudal end of the medulla to the rostral end of the mesencephalon (figs. 3 and 18). It is common to subdivide it into three portions: caudally the *nucleus of the spinal trigeminal tract* (nucleus tractus spinalis nervi trigemini), in the middle the *chief or principal sensory nucleus* (nucleus sensibilis principalis nervi trigemini) and rostrally the *mesencephalic nucleus* (nucleus mesencephalicus nervi trigemini).

The afferent, sensory, trigeminal fibres have their perikarya in the semilunar ganglion. Having entered the pons, they course in a dorsomedial direction and most of them dichotomize in a short ascending and a long descending branch. Some fibres run caudally without bifurcating. The mass of descending fibres constitute the *spinal trigeminal tract*[1] (tractus spinalis nervi trigemini), a distinct fibre bundle which is situated just underneath the lateral surface of the medulla oblongata (fig. 6), and a little deeper in the lower part of the pons (fig. 13) where it is covered by the fibres of the middle cerebellar peduncle (brachium pontis). The fibres of the tract continue in the rostralmost two segments of the cord in the zona terminalis. The fibres which are found in the spinal tract, as well as numerous collaterals, end in a longitudinal cell column medial to the tract, the *nucleus of the spinal trigeminal*

[1] The designation may be confusing, since it is common to use the term 'tract' (tractus) for fibre bundles connecting nuclei within the central nervous system, while the spinal trigeminal tract (as well as the solitary tract) is composed of the central processes of cells having their perikarya outside the central nervous system. In a similar way the fibres of the dorsal columns of the cord are axons from cells in the spinal ganglia.

tract (nucleus tractus spinalis nervi trigemini). This is caudally continuous with the pars gelatinosa of the dorsal horn and is composed of cells of different types. The axons of these mediate the further transmission of the sensory impulses. Long axons of the cells join the spinothalamic fibres (Walker, 1939), most of them crossed, and reach the medial part of the lateral thalamic nucleus (nucleus ventralis posteromedialis thalami). Sensory neurons of the third order conduct the impulses from the thalamus to the face region of the sensory cortex. Collaterals from the ascending fibres of the nucleus of the spinal trigeminal tract, and presumably also axons from some of its cells end in contact with cells in the reticular formation.

The *principal trigeminal nucleus* forms a rostral continuation of the nucleus of the spinal trigeminal tract, but has a somewhat different structure. Ascending fibres from this nucleus appear to join the fibres of the medial lemniscus.[1] The fibres from the principal nucleus do not cross the midline until they reach the mesencephalon (Russell, 1954), while those from the spinal nucleus cross shortly after their origin from the nucleus.[2]

The *mesencephalic trigeminal nucleus* (fig. 18) appears as a rostral continuation of the principal nucleus and forms a slender column of nerve cells a little lateral to the rostral part of the 4th ventricle and the cerebral aqueduct. The nucleus is composed of pseudounipolar cells like those in the sensory ganglia. It is not yet quite clear whether these cells, like those of the spinal ganglia, are derived from the neural crest (Pearson, 1949a, 1949b). The nucleus is accompanied by a distinct fibre bundle, the *mesencephalic root* (radix mesencephalica nervi trigemini) which is made up of ascending and particularly descending axons of the cells of the nucleus. Experimentally

[1] It is possible that the central trigeminal pathways in man are not exactly identical with those in animals (Smyth, 1939).

[2] Torvik (1957b) has shown that in the cat the principal sensory trigeminal nucleus gives off crossing as well as non-crossing ascending fibres, and that these two components come from different parts of the nucleus. If the same is true for man, some discordant findings in the literature may find a plausible explanation.

the descending fibres have been traced into the portio minor and into some branches of the trigeminal nerve.

Function

Extensive experimental and clinical investigations have demonstrated that the *three sensory trigeminal nuclei differ functionally* and mediate different kinds of somatic sensory impulses. The nucleus of the spinal trigeminal tract is related first and foremost to the transmission of impulses which are perceived consciously as pain and temperature, the principal nucleus to sensations of touch and the mesencephalic nucleus to proprioception.

Most of the fibres of the spinal trigeminal tract are thin. In man only about 10 per cent of them have diameters of 4 μ or more (Sjöqvist, 1938). As is well known, fibres transmitting impulses perceived as pain are commonly thin. The fibres in the spinal tract are distributed to the nucleus of the spinal tract in an orderly manner (fig. 18). The fibres of the ophthalmic nerve terminate most caudally, then follow the fibres of the maxillary nerve and rostral to these those of the mandibular nerve (Smyth, 1939; Harrison and Corbin, 1942). Furthermore the mandibular fibres are distributed most dorsally, then follow the maxillary fibres and most ventrally the ophthalmic fibres. The so-called medullary tractotomy of Sjöqvist (1938) for the treatment of trigeminal neuralgia is based on this pattern of distribution of the fibres. The procedure consists in transecting the spinal trigeminal tract by a superficial incision in the lowest part of the medulla, thus preventing the impulses in the descending fibres of the tract from reaching the nucleus.

Following this operation, pain sensibility in the homolateral half of the face is abolished, while the sense of touch is little affected. The perception of temperature suffers more or less. Further experiences with the operation have shown that the incision may be made more caudally than originally proposed by Sjöqvist (Olivecrona, 1942; White and Sweet, 1955). Thus only the caudalmost part of the spinal nucleus appears to be concerned in the transmission of pain perception. This may bear some relation to the fact that anatomically the nucleus may be subdivided into three parts, differing in structure (Olszewski, 1950). The histological structure of the caudal part resembles that of the dorsal horn. The middle levels appear to be related to temperature sensations (Smyth, 1939). An important advantage of the Sjöqvist operation is the preservation of the corneal reflex. Furthermore, there is no risk of a so-called 'neuroparalytic keratitis', an ulceration of the cornea which is commonly seen following operations for trigeminal neuralgia in which all afferent trigeminal fibres are transected. A comprehensive evaluation of the results of different operations for trigeminal neuralgia has recently been given by White and Sweet (1955).

The sense of touch is mediated by fibres which are somewhat thicker than those mediating pain, and the fibres which end in the principal nucleus are, in general, thicker than those to the spinal nucleus. This as well as clinical and experimental observations make it likely that impulses of touch are mediated chiefly by the principal nucleus.

However, it is scarcely safe to assume that the distinction between the functionally different parts of the trigeminal nucleus is sharp. Thus in experimental animals action potentials may be led off from the nucleus of the spinal tract following touch stimuli as well as pain stimuli, and following a medullary tractotomy touch sensibility is somewhat reduced. An anatomical feature which fits in with this view is the large number of fibres which dichotomize and give off one branch to the principal, another to the spinal nucleus, since it is unlikely that the same fibre may mediate sensations which are perceived as different sensory qualities.

Phylogenetic data and the central connexions of the two nuclei indicate that the spinal trigeminal nucleus is to be grouped with the grey of the dorsal horn in the spinal cord, the principal nucleus with the nuclei of the dorsal columns. When impulses of touch to some extent are mediated via the spinal nucleus, this is a parallel to the conduction of touch impulses in the spinothalamic tract (in addition to in the medial lemniscus). Following an interruption of the spinal trigeminal tract in man, the sense of pain is abolished also in the areas of supply of the intermediate, glossopharyngeal and vagus nerves (Brodal, 1947a).

As mentioned previously, sensory impulses which are propagated centrally through the trigeminal sensory nuclei may be depressed in their further conduction by influences from the cerebral cortex (see p. 25).

The conception that the mesencephalic trigeminal nucleus

is related to the transmission of proprioceptive sensibility rests on fairly solid ground. The peripheral, largely myelinated, fibres from its cells can, when degenerating, be followed into the muscular branches of the mandibular nerve (Szentágothai, 1948a; and others).

Some of the peripheral mesencephalic fibres, however, appear to run in sensory branches of the trigeminal nerve such as the alveolar nerves (Corbin, 1940) and are assumed to mediate sensations of pressure from the teeth and the peridontium. Action potentials can be led off from these nerves when pressure is applied to the teeth (Pfaffmann, 1939). It, therefore, appears likely that these fibres may be concerned in a mechanism which controls the force of the bite. Also some ordinary afferent trigeminal fibres run to the mesencephalic nucleus. The most convincing evidence that this nucleus is concerned in the mediation of proprioceptive sensations comes from investigations of the extrinsic eye muscles (see below p. 101) and from the recording of potentials in the nucleus on stretching of the masticatory muscles (Corbin and Harrison, 1940; Cooper, Daniel and Whitteridge, 1953a). Since the structure of the mesencephalic nucleus is in principle identical along its longitudinal extent, it appears likely that it is an entity also in a functional respect. The termination of some mesencephalic fibres in the cerebellum (Pearson, 1949b) fits in with the view of its function outlined above.[1]

Clinical Aspects

The trigeminal nerve has a twofold task. Its *motor functions* are examined by testing the masticatory muscles. A paresis or a paralysis of the temporal or masseter muscles can easily be ascertained by palpating the muscles when the patient tries to clench his jaws forcefully. In a peripheral (nuclear or infranuclear) affection the muscles will, furthermore, be flaccid and after some time become atrophic. The lateral, and to a lesser extent, the medial pterygoid muscles are tested by asking the

[1] It should be recalled in this connexion that the mesencephalic trigeminal nucleus is not a nucleus in the proper sense, but is to be compared with the sensory ganglia. It is possible, but has not so far been proved, that the impulses which are mediated via the mesencephalic nucleus and reach consciousness, have a relay in the principal sensory trigeminal nucleus.

patient to open his mouth. If these muscles on one side are paretic, the jaw will deviate to the affected side, because the paretic muscles will not, unlike their fellows on the other side, pull their half of the jaw forwards. The affection of the anterior belly of the digastric muscle and of the mylohyoid muscle is of relatively little importance, but may be recognized on careful palpation.

A *central, supranuclear trigeminal paresis*, due to damage to the corticofugal fibres acting on the motor nucleus, will not always betray itself clinically if the lesion is unilateral (for example in haemorrhages in the internal capsule). This is explained by the assumption that the motor trigeminal nucleus in most individuals receives a crossed as well as an uncrossed innervation from the cerebral cortex. However, a unilateral supranuclear paralysis is not infrequent (Monrad-Krohn, 1954). In pseudobulbar palsy (p. 33) there will be a bilateral supranuclear paralysis.

The *sensory functions of the trigeminal nerve* are examined by testing the response to touch, pain and temperature stimuli in its area of innervation. An *interruption of sensory trigeminal fibres* will produce a more or less marked sensory loss in the area of the affected branch. In lesions of the ophthalmic nerve the corneal reflex (reflex blinking on touching the cornea) will be abolished.

If the pathological process produces an *irritation of the nerve fibres*, pains are likely to appear in the area supplied by the fibres involved. Pains in the trigeminal area are most frequently met with as *trigeminal neuralgia*, characterized by paroxysms of severe pain which is localized to one half of the face, or, more frequently, to the area supplied by one of the major divisions. Frequently the paroxysms are provoked by stimuli to the skin or mucous membranes of the face, for example on chewing, on touching the skin of the face. In typical cases no loss of cutaneous sensation is present.

From experiences gained in surgical procedures for relieving the pain in trigeminal neuralgia it appears that the processes causing the pain paroxysms are not always situated peripheral to the ganglion or in it. In those cases in which no relief is obtained by medullary tractotomy, by transection of the root of the nerve or by injection of alcohol into the ganglion, it is assumed that a central disturbance of some kind is responsible for the symptoms.

Affections of the trigeminal nerve may be caused by a variety of pathological processes. To some extent the symptoms will vary, according to the site of the process. The *peripheral branches* may suffer in local processes of the face. It is important to be aware that the superior dental nerves may be involved in inflammations in the maxillary sinus (sinusitis). The *three chief divisions* may be affected by fractures of the skull passing through the foramina through which these nerves emerge. A motor loss will occur only in lesions of the mandibular nerve. Within the cranial cavity inflammations of the meninges and other processes may involve the trigeminal nerve. Of particular interest are morbid changes within the cavernous sinus, such as infraclinoid aneurysms of the internal carotid artery. If the aneurysm is situated high in the sinus it will affect primarily the ophthalmic nerve, if its position is lower, the other branches may also be involved (see fig. 15). On account of their neighbourhood, one or more of the nerves to the extrinsic eye muscles will frequently suffer simultaneously (see p. 105). The *semilunar ganglion* may be the seat of an inflammatory process. Just as in similar affections in other sensory ganglia, there will be pains and, usually somewhat later, vesicles in the skin and mucous membranes supplied by the nerve (*herpes zoster*). These symptoms are most frequently seen in the area of the ophthalmic nerve (herpes zoster ophthalmicus) with eruptions of vesicles in the skin of the forehead and on the cornea.[1] The fibres of the ophthalmic nerve are likewise particularly exposed in inflammations in the pneumatic cells in the apex of the pyramid of the temporal bone (petrositis, apicitis), which are usually propagated from an otitis. This is a consequence of the position of the ganglion

[1] The inflammation in herpes zoster appears to be due to a virus infection. Occasionally the inflammation may involve the motor root or the motor nucleus, with ensuing motor symptoms from the masticatory muscles.

on the apex of the pyramid (see Gradenigo's syndrome, p. 125).

Pathological processes in the *pons* may involve the trigeminal nerve or its nuclei. A pure motor loss may be seen in poliomyelitis or in progressive bulbar palsy. Vascular lesions, syringobulbia or inflammations will usually also affect the sensory trigeminal fibres or nuclei or the central ascending tracts from the latter. The considerable length of the sensory trigeminal nucleus, its subdivision into parts having different functions and the different course of the secondary sensory fibres from the spinal and principal sensory nuclei explain that there may be numerous variations in the symptomatology. Sensory symptoms due to central processes may be seen in affections of the thalamus.

The Abducent, Trochlear and Oculomotor Nerves

Anatomy

These cranial nerves, being numbers 6, 4 and 3, respectively, supply the external ocular muscles and the levator palpebrae muscle with *somatic efferent fibres*, and are thus the *motor nerves of the eyeball*. In addition the *oculomotor nerve* carries parasympathetic, *visceral efferent*, *fibres* to the smooth muscles of the eye. Since these nerves are closely related, both anatomically and functionally, it is practical to consider them together. First, however, an account of the peripheral course of each nerve will be given.

The *abducent nerve*, the 6th cranial nerve, leaves the brain stem as a thin bundle of fibres at the lower border of the pons, a little lateral to the pyramid (fig. 5). It runs ventrally and a little laterally in the pontine cistern and pierces the dura mater a little below and medial to the trigeminal nerve (fig. 15). It then continues its course in the cavernous sinus, where it is found lateral to the internal carotid artery and medial to the ophthalmic nerve (fig. 19). It enters the orbit through the superior orbital fissure and applies itself to the medial surface of the *lateral (external) rectus muscle* (musculus rectus oculi lateralis, s. temporalis). In the cavernous sinus the nerve is joined by some fibres from the sympathetic plexus on the internal carotid.

The *trochlear nerve*, the 4th cranial nerve, likewise is a slender fibre bundle. It is the only cranial nerve which leaves the brain stem on its dorsal side, namely just below the inferior colliculus (fig. 8). It then winds laterally around the rostral part of pons, continues in a ventral direction through the pontine cistern and penetrates the dura mater a little above the trigeminal nerve at the attachment of the tentorium cerebelli (fig. 15). Here the nerve enters the cavernous sinus, where it runs in a ventral direction above the abducent nerve and along the upper border of the ophthalmic nerve. It enters the orbit through the superior orbital fissure above the origin of the levator palpebrae muscle and continues in a ventral and medial direction to supply the *superior oblique muscle* (musculus obliquus oculi superior) from above (fig. 19). Some sympathetic fibres join the trochlear nerve in the cavernous sinus.

The *oculomotor nerve*, the 3rd cranial nerve, is the largest of the nerves to the external eye muscles, and is the only one of them which, in addition to somatic efferent, carries visceral efferent fibres. It emerges on the ventral side of the mesencephalon (fig. 5) in the interpeduncular fossa, medial to the cerebral peduncle, and runs in a ventral direction through the interpeduncular cistern. Usually it leaves the brain stem in the space between the posterior cerebral artery (above) and the superior cerebellar artery (below). The nerve pierces the dura as a round string lateral to the posterior clinoid process of the dorsum sellae (fig. 15) and enters the cavernous sinus, where it runs a little caudally in a ventral direction lateral to the internal carotid artery. In the anterior (ventral) part of the sinus it will thus be situated caudal (and medial) to the trochlear and abducent nerves. It enters the orbit below these nerves in the superior orbital fissure. In the orbit it subdivides into a superior and an inferior branch. The *ramus superior* runs lateral to the optic nerve and the ophthalmic artery and innervates (fig. 19) the *superior rectus muscle* (musculus rectus oculi superior) and the *levator palpebrae* (musculus levator palpebrae superioris). The *ramus inferior* is thicker than the upper branch and gives off short branches to the *inferior rectus muscle* (musculus rectus oculi inferior), the *medial rectus*

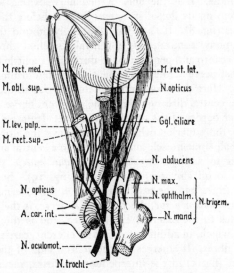

Fig. 19. The peripheral course of the nerves to the extrinsic eye muscles. (From Brodal, 1949.)

muscle (musculus rectus medialis) and a longer branch to the *inferior oblique muscle* (musculus obliquus inferior). From the latter branch some fibres pass to the ciliary ganglion (fig. 19). In this way the visceral efferent (parasympathetic, preganglionic) fibres of the oculomotor nerve reach the ciliary ganglion. The postganglionic fibres from this pass to the eyeball (p. 86). In the cavernous sinus the oculomotor nerve is joined by some sympathetic fibres.

The *somatic efferent fibres to the extrinsic eye muscles* are axons of large, multipolar nerve cells which are grouped in three nuclei, one for each of the nerves. They all belong to the medial column of motor nuclei which supplies musculature derived from the myotomes (fig. 3).

The *abducent nucleus*, the most caudal of these nuclei, is found in the pons, just underneath the floor of the 4th ventricle (fig. 13). As described previously (p. 69) the root fibres of the facial nerve make a bend dorsal to the nucleus. The fibres of the abducent nerve run in a ventral and slightly caudal direction (fig. 13) to their point of exit from the brain stem at the lower border of the pons.

The *trochlear nucleus* is situated at the level of the inferior colliculus, immediately ventral to the aqueduct of Sylvius. The medial longitudinal bundle runs immediately ventro-lateral to the nucleus (fig. 10). The root fibres of the nerve take a slightly caudal course and then cross the midline dorsal to the aqueduct to emerge on the surface below the inferior colliculus (fig. 8).

The *oculomotor nucleus* is found at the level of the superior colliculus, in a situation corresponding to that of the trochlear nucleus more caudally (fig. 10). The oculomotor nucleus is considerably larger than the abducent and trochlear nuclei. The medial longitudinal bundle is situated ventrolateral to the nucleus, which in cross-section has a triangular shape. It may be subdivided into a lateral and a medial part. The latter fuses with its fellow on the other side to an unpaired, median nucleus. The root fibres run in a ventral direction, medial to, and in part through, the red nucleus and emerge in the interpeduncular fossa as several bundles which fuse to form the trunk of the oculomotor nerve.

As in the other somatic efferent cranial nerve nuclei the cells in the oculomotor nucleus are arranged in groups according to the muscles which they supply. The most recent studies on this subject are those of Szentágothai (1942a) in the cat and Warwick (1953) in the monkey, and on most points they agree. The former author studied the effects of localized stimulations of small parts of the nucleus, the latter analysed the retrograde cellular changes which occur after extirpation of the individual extrinsic eye muscles. The regions of the nucleus supplying the various muscles appear to be arranged as columns of cells. When passing from rostrodorsal to ventrocaudal the muscles are represented in the following order: the inferior rectus, the inferior oblique, the medial rectus. The area of the superior rectus is found medial to those of the former two muscles (Warwick). The levator palpebrae has its representation most dorsocaudally. It is of interest that the latter muscle, unlike the others, is supplied by the oculomotor nucleus of both sides, since as a rule both upper eyelids are lifted simultaneously. Human cases showing paresis or paralysis of one extrinsic eye muscle only are rare, and even more rarely have histological studies been made in such cases. It is, therefore, no wonder that little is known concerning a possible localization within the oculomotor nucleus in man (for references see Warwick, 1953). However, it is fair to assume that conditions are in principle as in the monkey, even if some older observations seem to contradict this.

The *visceral efferent fibres in the oculomotor nerve* come from a particular nucleus, the *parasympathetic Edinger-Westphal nucleus*.[1] It is composed of cells which are smaller than those of the somatic efferent nucleus, and it is situated dorsomedial to the latter. The nucleus almost fuses in the midline with the nucleus of the other side. The fibres join the somatic efferent fibres in their peripheral course but leave the oculomotor nerve in the orbit to end in the ciliary ganglion (p. 85), in synaptical contact with its cells. Postganglionic fibres from the ganglion innervate the ciliary muscle and the pupillary sphincter.

The various *motor nuclei of the eye muscles are activated* (largely reflexly) by fibres from many sources. *Voluntary movements* of the eyes are initiated by fibres which come from the frontal lobe (area 8 in the inferior frontal gyrus) in front of the 'face' area in the motor region. The fibres follow the pyramidal tract. *Reflexly* the motor eye nuclei may be acted upon by impulses from three main sources: *optic impulses* via the optic nerve, *vestibular* via the medial longitudinal bundle, and *cortical* from the occipital lobe. The functional significance of these connexions will be dealt with in the chapter of the optic nerve. The following account will be restricted to the

[1] This has been doubted by some, but experimental studies (Warwick, 1954) have shown that practically all the cells of this nucleus send their axons to the ciliary ganglion.

peripheral pathways in the innervation of the extrinsic eye muscles.

The extrinsic eye muscles and their innervation present a number of interesting problems concerning the capacity of these muscles to produce extremely finely co-ordinated conjugate movements of the eyes. Several anatomical features are known which cast some light on the basis of this phenomenon. Thus the muscle fibres are thin and the motor units are small, that is: each nerve cell supplies only a few muscle fibres. This is in agreement with electromyographic studies of the extrinsic eye muscles in man (Björk and Kugelberg, 1953b). The vascular supply of the muscles is rich. Investigations undertaken in recent years have shown that the extrinsic eye muscles are amply provided with muscle spindles (as might be expected) and that the afferent impulses from these reach the mesencephalic trigeminal nucleus.

Contrary to what was generally believed previously, the extrinsic eye muscles in man contain a large number of muscle spindles, but they are smaller and have thinner capsules than the spindles in the skeletal muscles (Cooper and Daniel, 1949). (Strangely enough spindles appear to be absent in the extrinsic eye muscles in the cat and the monkey, while they are found in the goat.) On stretching of the extrinsic eye muscles action potentials can be led off from the mesencephalic trigeminal nucleus throughout its length (Cooper, Daniel and Whitteridge, 1953 a, b), and these potentials appear to come from the muscle spindles. In addition, action potentials of a longer latency can be obtained from other regions, such as the medial longitudinal bundle, the superior cerebellar peduncle and the superior colliculus. These potentials are assumed to have passed one or more synapses.

It is not yet decided along which routes the proprioceptive impulses from the extrinsic eye muscles reach the mesencephalic nucleus. Physiological studies (Cooper, Daniel and Whitteridge, 1951) indicate that at least some of them pass in the oculomotor nerve, in agreement with the anatomical finding that some fibres from the mesencephalic nucleus run peripherally in the nerves of the extrinsic eye muscles (Tarkhan, 1934). Possibly some proprioceptive fibres pass centrally in branches of the ophthalmic nerve.

Counts of the fibres in nerves to the extrinsic eye muscle in man (Björkman and Wohlfart, 1936) show that close to the brain stem the oculomotor nerve has some 24,000 fibres, the trochlear and the abducent nerves about 3400 and 6600, respectively. In all three nerves the diameters of the fibres vary, but considerable proportions of them have diameters of 3-6 μ and 8-11 μ. Conclusions as to whether some of the fibres are afferent cannot be made from these data.

Since proprioceptive impulses from the extrinsic eye muscles reach the mesencephalic trigeminal nucleus, presumably via fibres from its cells, and since fibres from this nucleus end also in the nuclei of the extrinsic eye muscles (Pearson, 1949a and others) it appears possible that there exists a two-neuron reflex arc which mediates stretch reflexes in these muscles (as is the case for the masticatory muscles). The problem of the proprioceptive innervation of the extrinsic eye muscles is, however, far more complex than it might appear from the simplified account given here, and there are still unsolved questions.

Function

The *task of the extrinsic eye muscles*, as is well known, is to produce the finely graded movements of the eyes which are necessary in order that the image of what we are looking at falls in the central fovea of the retina. This requires a very fine and harmonious control of the peripheral motor neurons, the axons of which form the 'final common path' for the impulses to the extrinsic eye muscles.

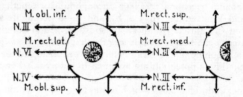

Fig. 20. Starling's diagram showing the actions of the extrinsic eye muscles.

In order to judge the function of the extrinsic eye muscles it is necessary to know the action of each of them. In a schematic way the action of the individual muscles may be shown as in the well-known diagram of Starling, reproduced in fig. 20. The arrows indicate the directions in which the various muscles are able to move the eyeball. It goes without saying that in conjugate movements of the eyes (p. 113) a simultaneous contraction of muscles belonging to both eyes is required, as well as a relaxation of their antagonists (reciprocal innervation). When, for example, a simultaneous contraction of the right lateral rectus and the left medial rectus moves both eyeballs to the right, the right medial and the left lateral recti will have to relax. In fact, however, conditions are far more complex since the action of an individual muscle varies according to the position of the eyeball in the orbit.

It will be seen from the diagram in the example mentioned above that the right superior and inferior oblique muscles will also have some effect in turning the right eye to the right, and the left superior and and inferior rectus muscles will assist in turning the left eye to the right side. This follows from the anatomical arrangement of the muscles. For example, the superior oblique, which has its attachment to the bulb behind its equator, will act as a lateral mover of the eyeball in all laterally directed positions of the eye, until in maximal abduction of the eye it will act as a pure rotator (when the axis of the muscle is in the equatorial plane). The superior rectus muscle will function as a pure elevator of the bulb only when the eye is slightly abducted, since only in this position is the axis of the muscle parallel to the longitudinal axis of the bulb. When the subject is looking straight ahead, the muscle will also to some extent act as an adductor and have a slight rotatory effect (see fig. 20). Thus, an apparently very simple movement such as looking to one side, involves several muscles on each side.

Electromyographic investigations of the human extrinsic eye muscles (Björk and Kugelberg, 1953 a, b) illustrate the features mentioned above. They show that there is activity, revealed as motor unit potentials, in the eye muscles in all positions of the eyes, except on maximal contraction of antagonists (for example in the lateral rectus when the eye bulb is turned maximally inwards). On looking straight ahead, all four recti muscles are active, but the activity in the individual muscles varies according to the position of the bulb. Studies like these illuminate the finely co-ordinated activity of the extrinsic eye muscles.

The *extrinsic eye muscles are examined* by testing the movements of the eyes in different directions. On account of the complex interplay between the muscles, it is not always an easy task to determine paresis or paralysis of a single muscle.

Furthermore, contractures in the non-paralysed muscles may in the course of time produce secondary changes. When one of the nerves is affected, however, as a rule characteristic changes appear: One of the eyes shows a squint (paralytic strabismus). In the beginning, the patient as a rule has diplopia and for this reason feels dizzy (vertigo). In *paralysis of the abducent nerve*, for example, the affected eye cannot be abducted fully. Some degree of movement of the eye in a lateral direction from the mid-position is, however, possible, because the superior and inferior oblique muscles have some abductor action and because the medial rectus will relax. On turning his eyes to the non-paralysed side the patient may achieve fusion of the images on the two eyes, and, therefore, soon gets accustomed to keeping his head turned towards the paralysed side. In *paralysis of the trochlear nerve* the effect of the superior oblique muscle will not be felt. The eye cannot be moved downwards and outwards. *Oculomotor paralysis*, if complete, will result in the eye being turned downwards and outwards, because the superior rectus muscle and the superior oblique muscle now are acting alone. The upper eyelid will be drooping, *ptosis*.[1] In a gradually developing oculomotor palsy, the paresis of the levator palpebrae muscle is regularly the first to appear.

An *affection of the oculomotor nerve* central to the departure of the branch to the ciliary ganglion will also interrupt the visceral efferent fibres to the pupillary sphincter and the ciliary muscle.[2] The pupil, therefore, will be larger (mydriasis) than that on the normal side (reduced tone in the sphincter and predominant action of the dilatator). The *light reflex*, constriction of the pupil when light enters the eye, and pupillary constriction on accommodation and convergence of the eyes

[1] It should be recalled that an affection of the sympathetic innervation of the eye as well will give a ptosis on account of the paralysis of the smooth tarsal muscle. There will also be a miosis, a small pupil, on account of a deficient dilatator pupillae. See p. 126, Horner's syndrome.

[2] According to Sunderland and Hughes (1946) the majority of the constrictor fibres for the pupil in the proximal part of the oculomotor nerve are found in its upper segment.

will be abolished, since the efferent link in the relevant reflex arcs will be interrupted. Accommodation will also be impossible.

Clinical Aspects

Palsies of the external eye muscles belong to the relatively common cranial nerve palsies, particularly lateral rectus nerve palsy. *Infranuclear palsies* may occur in fractures of the skull, pathological processes on the base of the skull, inflammations of the meninges (meningitis), tumours of the meninges or diseases in the orbit. Aneurysms of the internal carotid artery in the cavernous sinus (see p. 95) may involve one or more of the nerves to the extrinsic eye muscles. The seat of the aneurysm will decide which of the nerves will be affected first and whether, as is usually the case, the ophthalmic nerve will also be compressed. On account of their long free course in the cisterns, the nerves may be stretched when the brain or the brain stem is displaced.

Tumours, particularly in the temporal lobe, or an epidural haematoma, for example, may press the medial surface of the temporal lobe with the uncus and also the cerebral peduncle in a medial direction against the tentorium ('tentorial herniation'). This will produce a stretching of the *oculomotor nerve*. If the brain stem is pressed caudally, this nerve may be bent because the posterior cerebral artery runs above it (Sunderland and Bradley, 1953). The nerve of the other side may also be affected in this way, but as a rule later.

The *abducent nerve* may be affected when the brain stem is pressed caudally in cases with increased intracranial pressure. Anatomical studies (Sunderland, 1948) make it probable that this is usually due to traction on the nerve exerted by the anterior inferior cerebellar artery which as a rule runs just above it. Possibly a similar mechanism is responsible for the abducent nerve palsy which occasionally occurs following spinal anaesthesia. Inflammations of the pneumatic cells of the temporal pyramid may sometimes affect the abducent nerve (see p. 95).

In many cases of ocular nerve palsies no cause can be ascertained. These frequently transitory palsies, which commonly tend to recur, are usually labelled as being 'rheumatic'.

In some cases the further course of the disease has shown them to be due to an aneurysm on the internal carotid artery (ophthalmoplegic migraine). A final, peripheral affection of the extrinsic eye muscles which deserves mention, are the pareses in myasthenia gravis, which are related to chemical disturbances at the motor end plates (acetylcholine-cholinesterase effect). The early involvement of the extrinsic eye muscles in this disease may be related to their being constantly active (Björk and Kugelberg, 1953b).

Nuclear ocular nerve palsies may be seen in inflammations and tumours in the mesencephalon and/or pons, usually then combined with damage to other structures, particularly the pyramidal tract (see p. 125). A pure affection of the nuclei of ocular nerves occurs, for example, in poliomyelitis.[1] Chronic progressive ophthalmoplegia until recently was assumed to be due to a degeneration of the cells in the nuclei of the extrinsic eye muscles (see progressive bulbar palsy, p. 33). Recent histological studies of the eye muscles, however, show that at least in most of these cases there is a primary affection of the muscles of the type seen in progressive muscular dystrophies (Kiloh and Nevin, 1951; Schwarz and Liu, 1954; Nicolaissen and Brodal, 1959).

In the so-called *internal ophthalmoplegia* only the intrinsic smooth muscles of the eye are affected, in *external ophthalmoplegia* these are spared while the extrinsic muscles are paretic or paralytic. Presumably these types are due to an isolated affection of either the visceral efferent (Edinger-Westphal nucleus) or the somatic efferent oculomotor nucleus. Since the visceral efferent fibres run rather close together in the oculomotor nerve (Sunderland and Hughes, 1946) dissociated palsies of these types may also be seen in lesions which affect only the proximal part of the oculomotor nerve.

Supranuclear ocular nerve palsies will appear in lesions of the descending fibres to the nuclei from the cerebral cortex (the frontal and occipital lobes, see p. 114). In such cases both eyes will be affected, and consequently there will be disturbances of conjugate eye movements. These will be described in the

[1] In rare cases one of the nuclei only may be affected (Brodal, 1945).

following chapter. A particular disturbance of conjugate eye movements, nystagmus, has been considered above (p. 59).

The Optic Nerve

Anatomy

The 2nd cranial nerve, the optic nerve, is not a cranial nerve in the proper sense, but corresponds to a tract, since the retina

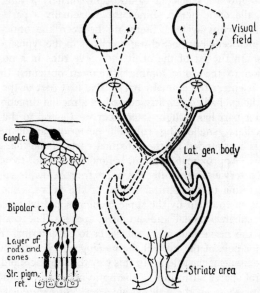

Fig. 21. Diagram of the path followed by the optic impulses in the retina (to the left) and in the central parts of the optic system.

develops from the optic cup. In man the optic nerve is made up of more than 1 million nerve fibres, i.e. some 38 per cent of all cranial nerve fibres (Bruesch and Arey, 1942). This numerical relation may be taken as a morphological expression of the functional importance of the optic nerve.

The optic nerve is formed by the central processes of the ganglion cells of the retina. These receive impulses from the bipolar cells, which again are activated by the sensory cells, the cone and rod cells, which react to light waves (fig. 21). The central processes (axons) of the ganglion cells converge in the innermost layer of the retina towards the optic disc (papilla nervi optici). This is situated a little medial to the posterior pole of the eyeball with the macula. When the nerve fibres have pierced the sclera in the optic disc they acquire myelin sheaths and are collected to an approximately 4 mm. thick string, the optic nerve. Since this is actually a part of the central nervous system, there are between the optic nerve fibres glial cells but no Schwann cells as in the typical cranial nerves. In the fat of the orbit the nerve runs in a posterior direction to the optic foramen (foramen opticum) through which it enters the cranial cavity. The first part of the nerve (near the eyeball) is slightly curved in a medial direction, the posterior part has a slight lateral curve. Lateral to the nerve is the ciliary ganglion (fig. 19). The posterior part of the optic nerve is surrounded by the proximal parts of the four rectus muscles. Approximately 1 cm. behind the eyeball the central retinal artery and vein enter the nerve from below, to continue to the retina in the central region of the nerve. The optic nerve is surrounded by the three meninges and by extensions of the subarachnoidal and subdural spaces. The pia mater covers the nerve and gives off septa to its interior. At the posterior pole of the eyeball the meninges fuse with the connective tissue of the sclera. In this way the subarachnoidal and subdural spaces surrounding the optic nerve end blindly. In the optic foramen the ophthalmic artery runs caudolateral to the nerve.

In its short intracranial course the optic nerve takes a medial direction and fuses with its fellow of the other side. In this way the *optic chiasm* (chiasma opticum), the crossing of the optic nerves (fig. 5), is formed. The chiasm is situated in the chiasmatic cistern (cisterna chiasmatis), above the sulcus chiasmatis of the sphenoid bone, in front of the sella turcica.

From the chiasm the axons of the optic nerve continue in a posterior (dorsâl) direction as the *optic tract* (tractus opticus), one on each side. The optic tract lies on the lateral surface of the cerebral peduncle, and can be followed into the *lateral geniculate body* (corpus geniculatum laterale). Most of the fibres of the optic nerve (and tract) end in synaptical contact with the cells of the lateral geniculate body. Others bend medially into the mesencephalon to the *superior colliculus* and the *pretectal region* (regio pretectalis). The nerve cells of the lateral geniculate body give off axons which run in the *optic radiation* (radiatio optica) to the striate area.[1]

The optic chiasm has important relations to some other structures. Lateral to it is the internal carotid artery (fig. 19). Behind it (dorsàlly) is the infundibulum and the hypophyseal stalk (fig. 5). The anterior cerebral artery runs from the internal carotid in a ventral direction above (rostral to) the optic nerve, while the ophthalmic artery, as mentioned above, runs below it. The topographical relations to the arteries may result in pressure on the optic nerve or chiasm when the arteries are the seat of aneurysms.

Of theoretical and practical interest is the existence of a marked *localization in the arrangement of the fibres from different parts of the retina in their course in the optic nerve, the chiasm, the optic tract, and further centrally*. First should be noticed the *partial crossing of fibres in the optic chiasm* (fig. 21). All fibres which come from the lateral (temporal) halves of the two retinae continue without crossing in the homolateral optic tract. Fibres from the medial (nasal) halves, however, cross in the chiasm to the optic tract of the contralateral side. As a consequence all light which enters the eyes from the *left* (and therefore impinges on the *right* halves of both retinae) gives rise to impulses which will be conducted centrally in the *right* optic tract and finally to the *right* striate area. (The limit in the retina goes vertically through the macula.) The localization is,

[1] The optic nerve also contains some efferent fibres to the eye. In the most posterior region of the chiasm there are, furthermore, some fibres which apparently have no relation to the optic system. They are called the supraoptic or hypothalamic commissure.

however, far more detailed. In the optic nerve the fibres are arranged largely according to their regions of origin within the retina, that is, fibres from the upper retinal quadrants are found in the upper part of the nerve, those from the lower in the lower, and macular fibres in the centre. In the optic tract

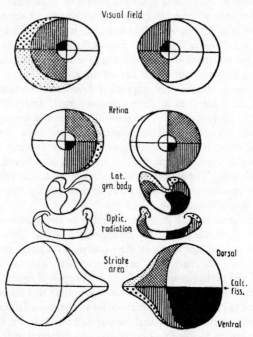

Fig. 22. Diagram of localization within the optic system. (From Brodal, 1943, redrawn from Poljak.)

both crossed and uncrossed fibres from the two homonymous (both right or both left) retinal halves will then meet, and fibres from corresponding points in the two retinae will run together. In the optic tract, however, a certain rearrangement of the fibre groups takes place, with the result that the fibres from the central parts of the retinae occupy a rather large part of its cross-sectional area above (rostrally) and laterally. The fibres from the lower parts of the retina are found laterally, those from the upper parts medially. The fibres end in the same pattern in the lateral geniculate body (fig. 22).

This localization is also preserved in the following link in the optic pathway, the *optic radiation*, which is formed by the axons of the cells in the lateral geniculate body and goes to the striate area (fig. 21). When leaving the lateral geniculate body this large fibre bundle makes a lateral and slightly ventral bend in the caudo-dorsal part of the internal capsule (its retrolenticular part), then swings in a posterior direction (dorsally) on the lateral side of the temporal and occipital horns of the lateral ventricle to the *striate area* (area striata, fig. 25). This is situated above and below (rostrally and caudally to) the calcarine fissure on the medial surface of the occipital lobe. In the striate area the fibres of the optic radiation end in a localized manner. Each small part of the retina will, therefore, be 'represented' in a particular small region in the striate area ('the cortical retina'). From fig. 22 it will be seen that the upper parts of the retina are 'represented' above the calcarine fissure, the lower parts below it, and that the central parts are found posteriorly, the peripheral ones anteriorly.

The localization within the optic system has been established by anatomical investigations. The arrangement of the fibres within the optic nerve and their pattern of termination in the lateral geniculate body has been determined by tracing the fibres which degenerate following lesions of the retina. Likewise the distribution of trans-neuronal changes in the lateral geniculate after localized lesions of the retina has given valuable information (Le Gros Clark and Penman, 1934). Following small lesions in the striate area, the ensuing retro-grade cell loss in the lateral geniculate body indicates those parts of the latter which send their axons to the damaged part in the cortex. The localization throughout the optic system has been synthesized by comparing the results of these two types of study. The conclusions arrived at have been confirmed by physiological experiments and clinical observations, by electrical stimulations and recordings and by studies of the consequences of lesions of the optic system in man.

From fig. 22 it will be seen that the small central regions of the retina are represented by a far larger area in the optic cortex (striate area) than the peripheral regions of the retina. This is what would be expected, since vision is sharpest in the macula. It is also in agreement with several features in the anatomical organization.

Thus in the retina the sensory cells are more densely packed and more slender in the macular region than more peripherally. Furthermore, there are in the macular regions many monosynaptic connexions, that is: one cone cell has connexions with one bipolar cell only, and one bipolar cell with one ganglion cell. More peripherally one ganglion cell collects impulses from many bipolar cells and one such cell from many sensory cells (Poljak, 1941). The association cells also have shorter processes in the central regions of the retina than in the peripheral.

The fusion of impulses from corresponding points in the two retinae appears to take place in the striate area, since crossing and non-crossing fibres are distributed to different layers of the 6-layered lateral geniculate body (Le Gros Clark and Penman, 1934; Glees and Le Gros Clark, 1941). Fibres from corresponding parts of these layers end in the same region of the striate area. This arrangement appears to be a morphological feature which makes possible a fusion of impulses from both eyes.

In the lateral geniculate body, each optic nerve fibre appears to have synaptical contact with 5 or 6 cells only (Glees and Le Gros Clark, 1941). In agreement with this the number of nerve cells in the lateral geniculate exceeds the number of optic nerve fibres. It has not yet been determined whether the optic nerve fibres from the peripheral parts of the retina have contact with more cells than fibres from the macular region, but this seems a likely assumption.

Function

The optic pathways via the lateral geniculate body to the cortex of the striate area (Brodmann's area 17) represent the route for those *optic impulses which reach consciousness*. For the interpretation of the optic impressions it is also necessary that the regions around the striate area on the convexity of the hemisphere (Brodmann's areas 18 and 19) are intact. These areas are mutually interconnected by association fibres.

Optic impulses may also elicit reflexes. Here only some simpler optic reflexes will be considered, in which the efferent link in the reflex arc is formed by somatic or visceral efferent fibres in the nerves to the eye muscles.[1] *Under normal conditions the reflexly elicited eye movements are always conjugate,* that is: the two eyes are moved in parallel or in a slightly convergent position, in a manner which ensures that the axes of the two eyes meet in the point at which the subject is looking. As mentioned above (p. 103) movements of this type require a finely graded innervation of the various extrinsic eye muscles. The afferent links in the arcs for simpler optic reflexes are formed by optic nerve fibres which leave the optic tract and enter the mesencephalon. (Other optic reflexes may be elicited from the vestibular apparatus (see p. 59) and from the muscles of the neck.) The afferent optic reflex fibres end partly in the superior colliculus, partly in the so-called pretectal region, situated ventral to the former. Within the colliculus the fibres display a localization in their distribution. This has been shown by anatomical studies, and has also been confirmed physiologically (see Cooper, Daniel and Whitteridge, 1953c). Each part of the retina is 'represented' in a particular region of the *superior colliculus.* This may be considered a lower reflex centre regulating the conjugate eye movements which occur as a response to optic stimuli. The centre may be influenced from the cerebral cortex.

Electrical stimulation of small spots in the superior colliculus produces conjugate eye movements. The animal's eyes are directed to that point in the surroundings, the representation of which is in the stimulated part of the colliculus (Apter, 1945, 1946). For example, stimulation of an area of the colliculus which corresponds to a point in the surroundings below and to the left will produce movements of the eyes which direct the gaze to this point. Also movements of the head and trunk, mediated by descending fibres from the superior colliculus, will take part in such reflex actions. Presumably proprioceptive impulses from the extrinsic eye muscles (p. 101) are also involved in such reflexes (Cooper, Daniel and Whitteridge, 1953 a, b).

The superior colliculus is connected with the motor nuclei

[1] A more complete account of optic reflexes may be found in Brodal (1948).

supplying the extrinsic eye muscles by fibres which mediate the finely graded innervation of these muscles. In spite of many studies the anatomy of these connexions is not yet fully known. In man the reflex functions of the superior colliculus are to a larger extent than in lower mammals under the *control of higher cortical reflex centres in the occipital lobe* (areas 17, 18 and 19). Electrical stimulation of these regions can produce conjugate eye movements in all directions, most easily in the horizontal plane, in man (Penfield and Rasmussen, 1950, and others) and in monkeys (Crosby, 1953, and others). Fibres appear to run from those parts which on stimulation produce movements in a certain direction to the corresponding region in the superior colliculus (Crosby and Henderson, 1948). (Possibly the connexions with the vestibular nuclei and the medial longitudinal bundle are also of importance for these cortical reflexes.) It appears that the occipital area for eye movements is related to those reflex movements of the eyes which make possible the *fixation of the gaze* (necessary, for example in reading). This area presumably is acted upon by association fibres from other parts of the cerebral cortex. Converging movements of the eyes when the gaze is fixed at close objects, likewise appear to be elicited from the occipital 'centre'.

Conjugate eye movements can also be elicited from the frontal lobe (particularly the area 8) on electrical stimulation in man and animals. The efferent fibres appear to follow those of the pyramidal tract and to terminate in relation to the nuclei of the nerves to the eye muscles.[1] Clinical data make it appear likely that *voluntary movements of the eyes* are mediated via these connexions.

[1] On the basis of anatomical investigations of the terminal regions of the corticomesencephalic fibres and stimulation experiments Szentágothai (1943b) maintains that the corticofugal fibres from the frontal region end in the small interstitial nucleus of Cajal in the mesencephalon, at the level of the oculomotor nucleus. This nucleus also is thought by him to represent the 'gaze centre' for vertical and rotatory movements of the eyeballs. The 'gaze centre' for horizontal movements is assumed to be situated in the reticular formation, lateral to the interstitial nucleus.

However, impulses entering the brain in the optic nerve do not only elicit reflexes which involve the external eye muscles. The smooth muscles of the eye may also be activated in this way, namely in changes of the size of the pupils and in accommodation.

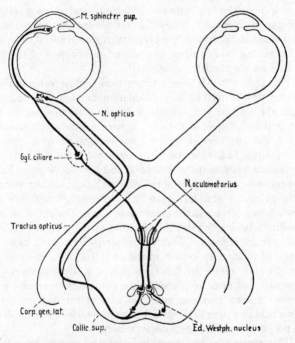

Fig. 23. A simplified diagram of the reflex arc for the light reflex.
(From Brodal, 1949.)

The *light reflex*, constriction of the pupil when light enters the eye, is mediated by a reflex arc in which the afferent link is represented by optic nerve fibres to the superior colliculus (fig. 23). The efferent link is formed by visceral efferent fibres from the Edinger-Westphal nucleus and postganglionic neurons of the ciliary ganglion with their axons to the pupillary sphincter. The central connexions in the reflex arc are not known exactly, but since pupillary constriction occurs on both eyes if light is thrown into one eye (consensual reaction), afferent optic impulses must reach the Edinger-Westphal nucleus of both sides. Secondary fibres cross, in part at least, in the posterior commissure (Magoun and Ranson, 1935; Szentágothai, 1942b). The *reflex 'centre'* does not appear to be in the colliculus, but in the pretectal region, ventral to it, because among other things, an isolated destruction of the colliculi does not abolish the light reflex.

This light reflex is purely subcortical.[1] However, pupillary constriction as well as accommodation can also be produced from the cortical occipital eye field. In man this part of the cerebral cortex appears to be the 'centre' for the *accommodation reflex*, the adaption of the eyes for looking at near objects. The afferent link is formed by the optic pathways via the lateral geniculate body to the striate area, and corticocollicular fibres appear to be the first part of the efferent link of the arc, visceral efferent fibres the last (pre- and postganglionic, via the oculomotor nerve and the ciliary ganglion). The act of accommodation is closely related to fixation of the gaze, which as a rule occurs reflexly. This *fixation reflex* likewise must be assumed to have its 'centre' in the occipital lobe. In order for the fixation reflex to function properly, it appears to be essential that optic impressions are consciously perceived. It is well known that our attention to and interest in certain objects in our surroundings determines which of these will act as proper stimuli for the fixation reflex.

The various reflexes are functionally closely bound together. Thus on looking at close objects, the accommodation

---

[1] According to recent investigations the size of the pupil in most mammals and in man appears to be determined mainly by varying tone in the sphincter pupilli muscle. The dilatator muscle, the existence and importance of which have been doubted, appears to be of less importance. There is good evidence that the pupillary dilatation following stimulation of the sympathetic fibres to the eye is, at least chiefly, due to a constriction of the vessels of the iris.

reflex and the fixation reflex will be accompanied by a reflex constriction of the pupils.

The *function of the optic nerve* is examined by testing the visual acuity and the visual field. In the latter examination it is important to determine not only the extent of the visual field in all directions, but also to decide by perimetry whether there are 'blind spots' in the visual field.[1] An important supplementary examination is ophthalmoscopy. This gives information on the appearance of the fundus of the eye (haemorrhages, exudations, choked discs, papilloedema and other pathological changes). Testing of the light reflex may give important information (see below). Among other methods of examination may be mentioned testing of the optokinetic nystagmus (nystagmus produced by optic stimuli, for example alternating light and dark stripes on a revolving drum).

Clinical Aspects

On account of the length of the optic pathways and their special organization a careful examination of visual functions may give important diagnostic information. An *interruption of one optic nerve* will result in complete blindness of the corresponding eye. The light reflex, when tested by illumination of the blind eye, will be absent on both eyes, while it can be elicited on both eyes if light is thrown into the sound one, provided that the efferent link in the reflex arc (the visceral efferent oculomotor fibres) is intact. This is explained by the course of the optic nerve fibres in the mesencephalon (fig. 23). In a partial lesion of the optic nerve (meningeomas arising from the dura of the lesser wing of the sphenoid, aneurysms on the anterior cerebral artery) information of the site of the lesion can be obtained by examining the visual fields. This is due to the topical arrangement of the fibres in the optic nerve (see p. 110). *Lesions of the optic chiasm* will produce typical defects in

---

[1] The physiological 'blind spot', which is due to the absence of sensory cells in the part of the retina covering the optic papilla, as is well known, is not perceived normally, because the 'spots' on the two eyes are not corresponding.

the visual fields. If the crossing fibres are interrupted (hypophyseal tumours) vision is lost in the temporal halves of both visual fields: *bitemporal hemianopsia* (fig. 24B). An interruption of the lateral, uncrossed fibres (aneurysms on the internal carotid) results in defects in the medial part of the visual field

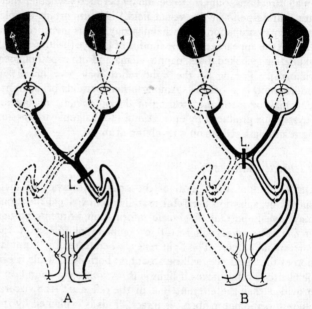

Fig. 24. Diagrams of the visual field defects following a lesion of the optic tract (A) and of the optic chiasm (B). (From Brodal, 1949.)

of the eye on the affected side. In *lesions of the optic tract* (fig. 24A) the conduction of impulses from the halves of both retinae on the side of the lesion will be interrupted. There will be a defect in the contralateral halves of both visual fields: *homonymous hemianopsia*. A defect of this type will, however, also occur in a total interruption of the optic pathways at any site central to the optic chiasm, for example in a *destruction of the lateral geniculate body, of the optic radiation or of the entire striate area.* Such lesions may be caused by tumours in, or traumata to, the occipital lobe, but it is important to recall that on account of the course taken by the fibres of the optic radiation, lesions in the temporal lobe may also produce homonymous visual field defects. On account of the size of the optic radiation and the striate area, lesions of these will frequently be only partial. The sharp localization within the optic system explains why in such lesions there will be only limited defects (scotomata) in the corresponding regions of the homonymous halves of the visual fields. A mapping of the scotomata by means of perimetry permits an exact determination of the site of the lesion. In lesions central to the lateral geniculate body the light reflex (direct and consensual) will be preserved, since its reflex arc (p. 115) is not involved. In lesions of the optic tract the light reflex can be elicited only from the functioning halves of the two retinae. In lesions which produce an irritation of the striate area or its neighbouring cortex, the patient may experience subjective visual phenomena, for example as an initial symptom in epileptic seizures arising in this part of the cortex (Penfield and Kristiansen, 1951).

Lesions of the superior colliculus and the pretectal region may leave the pathway for optic impulses to the cortex intact, but may result in disturbances in those optic reflexes which have their 'centres' in this region. Thus paralysis of gaze may be seen (the conjugate eye movements in one or more directions may be abolished), for example in tumours of the pineal body. In agreement with the 'representation' of the various parts of the retina in the superior colliculus (the lower retinal regions are 'represented' above and medially in the colliculus) in the beginning usually a paresis of upward conjugate movements (the pressure acts from above) is found (Müller and Wohlfart, 1947).

Pareses of gaze may occur also in *lesions of the cortical eye fields.* In lesions of the frontal eye field (area 8) the patient may be unable to move his eyes *voluntarily* to the opposite side. He may, however, be able to follow with his eyes an object moving in all directions if it is moved slowly, and he will be able to read. This is assumed to be due to integrity of the occipital eye field and the functioning of the fixation reflex (Holmes, 1938). If this cortical area is damaged, however, there will be difficulties in fixing objects with the eyes, even if the eyes can be moved voluntarily. Accommodation will also suffer. Both cortical eye fields (frontal and occipital) appear to be necessary for a perfect functioning of the eyes.

A peculiar phenomenon is the so-called *Argyll Robertson* sign: abolished pupillary reaction to light, but preserved accommodation reflex. It is seen most frequently in syphilis of the central nervous system (see p. 124). In spite of many attempts, it has not yet been possible to explain how the dissociation between those two reflexes is produced. (Some relevant literature in Brodal, 1948.)

The Olfactory Nerve

Anatomy

The olfactory nerve, the 1st cranial nerve, is formed by some 20 small bundles of nerve fibres which enter the under surface of the olfactory bulb. They penetrate the cribriform plate of the ethmoid bone and are distributed to the upper part of the nasal cavity on the superior nasal concha and to the upper part of the nasal septum facing this. In this 'area olfactoria' the nasal mucosa has a yellowish tint.

The olfactory fibres are considered as being *visceral afferent*. Contrary to other visceral afferent fibres, they are not cell processes of ganglion cells, but are central, unmyelinated processes of the olfactory sensory cells. The latter are slender cylindrical epithelial cells provided with sensory hairs and are surrounded by supporting cells. Where the fibre bundles pass through the cribriform plate, they are covered by extensions from the meninges. In this way the subarachnoid space is related to the lymphatic vessels in the nasal cavity, enabling infections from the nose to spread intracranially.

In the *olfactory bulb* (bulbus olfactorius, fig. 5) the olfactory fibres establish synaptical contact with the dendrites of the mitral cells, which send their axons centrally in the *olfactory tract* (tractus olfactorius), but other cells in the olfactory bulb also take part in the conduction of olfactory impulses. The fibres of the olfactory tract continue in its prolongations, the lateral and medial olfactory striae (stria olfactoria lateralis and medialis) on either side of the olfactory trigone (trigonum olfactorium) and the anterior perforated space (substantia

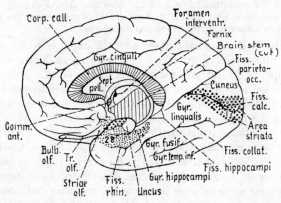

Fig. 25. The medial surface of the right cerebral hemisphere. The primary olfactory cortex is indicated by coarse stippling. (From Brodal, 1949.)

perforata anterior). The *terminal areas of the olfactory fibres* have been determined in experimental investigations, by cutting the olfactory tract and mapping the ensuing terminal degeneration in the monkey (Meyer and Allison, 1949) and the rabbit (Le Gros Clark and Meyer, 1947). In man the terminal areas appear to correspond to those in the monkey (Allison, 1954). The majority of the fibres end in the anterior (ventral) part of the *uncus* (fig. 25), which appears to be the most important part of the *primary cortical olfactory area* in man. Other fibres pass to the posterior part of the orbital cortex (the prepiriform area) and some to the anterior perforated space.

Experimentally, fibres have, furthermore, been traced to some small nuclei, among them the phylogenetically old, medial part of the amygdaloid nucleus.

For the other forms of sensation, a primary sensory cortex, receiving the sensory impulses, is surrounded by a secondary sensory sphere, which appears to be necessary for the proper interpretation of the sensory impressions. By way of analogy, it might be surmised that the cortex adjoining the primary olfactory cortex, the entorhinal area (Brodmann's area 28, fig. 25), represents a secondary olfactory area. This assumption (Brodal, 1947b) is, however, contradicted by the results of experimental studies by Adey and Meyer (1952), since these authors were unable to find any fibre connexions from the primary olfactory cortex to the entorhinal area.

The further central pathways for the impulses which reach the primary olfactory cortex appear to be multifarious and complicated, and are not yet known in detail. Following electrical stimulation of the olfactory bulb action potentials may be led off from numerous structures in the brain, among them the hippocampus (Berry, Hagamen and Hinsey, 1952). The traditional conception that the hippocampus is a part of the brain especially related to the sense of smell, can, however, not be upheld (see Brodal, 1947b, for a review). An increasing number of observations indicate that this peculiar structure may bear some relation to emotional processes and complex psychic functions (see for example Kaada, Jansen and Andersen, 1953).

In man the sense of smell and the olfactory apparatus is rudimentary as compared with those of many animals. In spite of this, the hippocampus (with the fornix) and the cingulate gyrus (fig. 25) which are mutually interconnected, are particularly well developed in man. These, as well as other morphological features argue strongly against assuming a closer relation between the sense of smell and the hippocampus. Olfactory impressions, in addition to their role in conscious perception, are important stimuli for a series of reflexes, particularly reflexes related to nutrition and reproduction.

Function

The olfactory nerve is examined by letting the patient try to identify the smell of various substances. Each side of the nose is tested separately. Substances which will produce an irritation of the nasal mucosa (as for example ammonia) must be avoided, since the trigeminal stimulation which occurs, may be misinterpreted by the patient as an olfactory sensation. A more exact determination of the sense of smell may be obtained by Elsberg's method, quantitative olfactometry (Elsberg and Levy, 1935; Kristensen and Zilstorff-Pedersen, 1953).

Clinical Aspects

A reduced or abolished sense of smell on one or both sides may be met with in pathological processes which damage the olfactory tract or bulb, such as fractures of the skull, tumours and inflammations in the anterior cranial fossa. The results of any examination of the sense of smell must be evaluated critically, since local alterations in the mucosa (a common cold!) or narrow nasal passages (nasal stenosis) may produce a reduction of olfactory acuity.

Uncinate fits are a peculiar phenomenon which deserve mention. Short-lasting olfactory sensations (most frequently of an unpleasant character), occurring in the absence of objective olfactory stimuli, are accompanied by some slight degree of reduced consciousness, for example of a feeling that the surroundings appear distant or dim. Sometimes involuntary smacking, chewing or licking movements are seen. Uncinate fits, which may herald a regular epileptic fit, are assumed to be due to pathological processes in the region of the uncus. This view gains considerable support from the observation that electrical stimulation of the uncus in conscious human beings may elicit an uncinate fit (Penfield and Kristiansen, 1951).

The Terminal Nerve

The *nervus terminalis* is a small bundle of nerve fibres which runs from the region of the medial olfactory stria, medial to the anterior perforated space, through the cribriform plate to the nasal septum. When the old anatomists counted the cranial nerves, the terminal nerve remained unrecognized and, therefore, has got no number. Topographically and possibly also functionally, it has relations to the olfactory nerve. It is rudimentary in man and higher mammals, but can be found at foetal stages. It possesses a small ganglion and contains afferent and efferent fibres (Pearson, 1941). The terminal nerve is of no practical but of some theoretical interest.

Together with the terminal nerve run some fibres, the *vomeronasal nerve*, which come from the so-called organ of Jacobsohn (organon vomeronasale). This is situated on the nasal septum and contains sensory cells. Centrally these fibres have connexions with an accessory olfactory bulb. In man this, as well as the organ of Jacobsohn, becomes rudimentary even during foetal life (Humphrey, 1940).

Appendix

Some common syndromes

Adie's syndrome. This designation is used when the following constellation of symptoms appear in an otherwise normal person: Abolished patellar reflexes and pupils which react slowly and weakly to light but react on accommodation, although slowly. When such pupillary changes, which may be unilateral, occur alone, one often speaks of pupillotonia. The cause of the syndrome is unknown, but it bears no relation to syphilis of the central nervous system and is not to be confused with the Argyll Robertson sign.

Argyll Robertson sign. This is seen most frequently in syphilis of the nervous system, particularly in tabes dorsalis (locomotor ataxia), but may occur occasionally also in other diseases, such as epidemic encephalitis, disseminated sclerosis, syringobulbia, tumours of the pineal body (Müller and Wohlfart, 1947), of the superior colliculus or the 3rd ventricle. The Argyll Robertson pupil is a small pupil which does not react to light but reacts briskly on accommodation (see p. 120).

Bell's phenomenon. When a patient suffering from a peripheral facial palsy attempts to close his eyes, it can be seen that the eyeballs move upward and slightly outward (contraction of the superior rectus muscle, relaxation of the inferior rectus). The same movement of the eyeballs occurs normally on closing the eyes, but it becomes visible only when the upper lid cannot be lowered, such as in a peripheral facial palsy (paresis of the orbicularis oculi muscle).

Benedikt's syndrome is the designation used for the following combination of symptoms: Unilateral oculomotor palsy (p. 104) and hyperkinesias and pareses on the contralateral side of the body. The ocular symptoms are caused by damage to the fibres of the oculomotor nerve in the brain stem. The hyperkinesias are attributed to a concomitant affection of the red nucleus or neighbouring structures. (Some of the oculomotor fibres pass through the red nucleus, p. 99.) The cause of the symptoms may be a vascular lesion, less frequently a tumour. Depending on the extension of the lesions other symptoms may also occur (see for example Kristiansen, 1940).

Crocodile-tears, syndrome of: Secretion of tears on eating or on stimuli producing secretion of saliva. This phenomenon may appear in later stages of peripheral facial palsies due to a lesion central to the geniculate ganglion and is explained on the basis of erroneous regeneration of nerve fibres (Taverner, 1955). Fibres of the intermediate nerve which have originally supplied salivatory glands on regeneration enter the Schwann sheaths belonging to fibres having innervated the lacrimal gland.

Foster Kennedy's syndrome. Unilateral blindness or larger scotomas accompanied by atrophy of the optic disc and anosmia on the same side and a choked disc on the other eye. The syndrome may appear in basally situated tumours in the anterior cranial fossa (most frequently meningeomas) which produce a pressure atrophy of the optic and olfactory nerves on the same side and concomitantly an increase of intracranial pressure.

Foville's syndrome. Unilateral facial palsy and paralysis of conjugate eye movements to the same side, combined with a contralateral hemiplegia, due to a lesion in the pons. The pyramidal tract is involved above its crossing. The lesion affects the facial and abducent nerves, but since there is a paralysis of conjugate eye movements to the affected side the ocular symptoms cannot be explained as being due to a unilateral damage to the abducent nerve only. The paralysis of gaze is commonly assumed to be caused by the involvement of a pontine gaze centre. (Some authors speak of a Foville syndrome even if there is only a unilateral abducent palsy, but no paralysis of gaze.)

Gradenigo's syndrome. A combination of pain in the area of the trigeminal nerve, usually in that of the 1st division (p. 95) and an abducent nerve palsy (p. 105). It is most commonly caused by an inflammation in the pneumatic cells in the pyramid of the temporal bone (petrositis, apicitis). (Above the apex of the pyramid the semilunar ganglion is found, and the abducent nerve courses close to this.)

Horner's syndrome. A combination of miosis (constricted pupil), ptosis (drooping of the upper lid) and enophthalmos (the eyeball being situated deeper in the orbit than normally). According to many investigators there is no real enophthalmos, but it appears to be present on account of the ptosis. The miosis is due to an interruption of sympathetic fibres to the dilatator pupilli muscle (prevalent action of the sphincter pupilli), the ptosis is caused by an interruption of the sympathetic fibres to the smooth tarsal muscle (m. tarsalis superior). This ptosis should not be confused with the ptosis occurring in a palsy of the oculomotor nerve (p. 104). A distinguishing feature is the widened pupil (mydriasis) in the latter case. Horner's syndrome may follow interruption of the axons of the postganglionic neurons in the sympathetic path to the eye (perikarya in the superior cervical ganglion). It may be seen, however, also in lesions of the sympathetic trunk above and including the stellate ganglion, where the preganglionic fibres from Th_{1-2} (ciliospinal centre) enter the sympathetic trunk. Finally it may follow lesions of the spinal cord at this level or more cranially, or lesions of the lateral part of the brain stem, since fibres from higher centres descend this way to reach the preganglionic sympathetic neurons of the intermediolateral cell column. On account of the interruption of the sympathetic fibres to the sweat glands, sweat secretion is frequently reduced in the homolateral half of the face in Horner's syndrome.

Marcus-Gunn phenomenon. On movements of the jaw there appear involuntary contractions of the upper eyelid. The phenomenon is assumed to be due to a congenital faulty innervation. Similar involuntary movements may be seen in the course of a peripheral facial palsy, as an expression of erroneous regeneration of fibres: Fibres originally destined for the orbicularis oris and other muscles around the mouth during regenerating have entered Schwann sheaths which run to the orbicularis oculi muscle. In movements of the mouth (speech, laughter, etc.) blinking and involuntary twitchings appear.

Millard-Gubler's syndrome. Facial palsy combined with a crossed hemiplegia, resulting from a focal lesion in the pons which involves the pyramidal tract on one side above its crossing. As in the many other types of so-called alternating hemiplegia (hemiplegia alternans: combination of a unilateral hemiplegia with a lesion of one of the cranial nerves on the opposite side) most commonly other symptoms are found in addition, indicating a damage to other nuclei, tracts or nerves. (Particularly in French literature, the various types of hemiplegia alternans are named after certain authors who first described them.) In the Millard-Gubler syndrome, frequently the abducent nerve will be affected on the same side as the facial (see above, Foville's syndrome). It may also often be combined with symptoms due to involvement of the trigeminal nerve, ascending sensory tracts or with cerebellar symptoms produced by an affection of the middle cerebellar peduncle. The lesion is most commonly of vascular origin.

Ramsay Hunt's syndrome. A combination of a peripheral facial palsy, with herpetic eruptions on the tympanic membrane, in the external auditory meatus and the concha of the auricle (most frequently also neuralgic pains in the same region). The herpetic eruptions and the pain are due to an inflammation in the geniculate ganglion where the afferent fibres of the intermediate nerve have their perikarya (p. 66). See also p. 79 and herpes zoster ophthalmicus (p. 95).

Sinus cavernosus syndrome. Oedema of the conjunctiva, the eyelids and the skin on the base of the nose with protrusion of the eyeball and paresis or paralysis of the oculomotor (p. 104), trochlear (p. 104) and abducent nerves (p. 104). All symptoms can be explained as being due to a thrombosis in the cavernous sinus (p. 80).

Wallenberg's syndrome. This name is used for a constellation of symptoms which is commonly seen following an occlusion of the posterior inferior cerebellar artery. This artery supplies the caudal parts of the cerebellar hemisphere and in addition gives off numerous small branches to the lateral part of the medulla dorsal to the inferior olive. As a rule there is a homolateral paresis of the tongue, pharynx and larynx (affection of root fibres of the hypoglossal, glossopharyngeal and vagus nerves, see fig. 6), loss of the sense of pain and temperature in the opposite half of the body (interruption of the spinothalamic tract), homolateral loss of pain and temperature sensibility in the face (affection of the spinal trigeminal tract and its nucleus), a homolateral Horner's syndrome (see p. 126, interruption of descending fibres to the ciliospinal centre), homolateral disturbances in co-ordination and a tendency to fall in the same direction (affection of the cerebellum).

Weber's syndrome. Combination of an oculomotor palsy with a hemiplegia on the opposite side. This syndrome may be produced by a lesion of the cerebral peduncle which encroaches upon the fibres of the oculomotor nerve.

References

Chiefly references to more recent literature are listed below. References to older works will be found in those cited.

Monographs

Brodal, A.: Nevro-anatomi i relasjon til klinisk nevrologi. Johan Grundt Tanum, Oslo 1943.
—— Centralnervesystemet, dets bygning og trekk av dets funksjon. Johan Grundt Tanum, Oslo, 1949. 2nd revised edition 1963.
—— Neurological Anatomy in Relation to Clinical Medicine. Clarendon Press, Oxford 1948. Reprinted 1952.
—— The Reticular Formation of the Brain Stem. Anatomical Aspects and Functional Correlations. William Ramsay Henderson Trust Lecture. Oliver & Boyd, Edinburgh 1957.
Brodal, A., O. Pompeiano and F. Walberg: The Vestibular Nuclei and their Connections. Anatomy and Functional Correlations. William Ramsay Henderson Trust Lecture. Oliver & Boyd, Edinburgh 1962.
De Jong, R. L.: The Neurologic Examination. Hoeber, New York 1950.
Monrad-Krohn, G. H.: The Clinical Examination of the Nervous System. 10th edition. H. K. Lewis & Co., Ltd., London 1954.
Olszewski, J. and D. Baxter: Cytoarchitecture of the Human Brain Stem. S. Karger, Basel 1954.
Penfield, W. and T. C. Erickson: Epilepsy and Cerebral Localization. A Study of the Mechanism, Treatment and Prevention of Epileptic Seizures. Charles C. Thomas, Springfield, Ill. 1941.
—— *W. and K. Kristiansen:* Epileptic Seizure Patterns. Charles C. Thomas, Springfield, Ill. 1951.
—— *and Th. Rasmussen:* The Cerebral Cortex of Man. Macmillan Comp., New York 1950.
Poljak, S. L.: The Retina. University of Chicago Press, Chicago 1941.
Sjöqvist, O.: Studies on pain conduction in the trigeminal nerve. Acta Psychiat. Neur., Suppl. *17:* 1-139, 1938.
Szentágothai, J.: Die Rolle der einzelnen Labyrinthrezeptoren bei der Orientation von Augen und Kopf im Raume. Akadémiai Kiadó, Budapest 1952.

Vraa-Jensen, G. Fr.: The Motor Nucleus of the Facial Nerve. E. Munksgaard, Köbenhavn 1942.

White, J. O. and W. H. Sweet: Pain. Its Mechanisms and Neurosurgical Control. Charles C. Thomas, Springfield, Ill. 1955.

Original Papers

Adey, W. R. and M. Meyer: Hippocampal and hypothalamic connexions of the temporal lobe in the monkey. Brain 75: 358-384, 1952.

Adrian, E. D.: Discharges from vestibular receptors in the cat. J. Physiol. 101: 389-407, 1943.

Allison, A. C.: The secondary olfactory areas in the human brain. J. Anat. 88: 481-488, 1954.

Alphin, Th. H. and W. T. Barnes: The course of the striae medullares in the human brain. J. Comp. Neur. 80: 65-68, 1944.

Andersen, P., J. C. Eccles and T. A. Sears: Presynaptic inhibitory actions. Presynaptic inhibitory action of cerebral cortex on the spinal cord. Nature 194: 740-741, 1962.

Apter, J. T.: Projection of the retina on superior colliculus of cats. J. Neurophysiol. 8: 123-134, 1945.

—— Eye movements following strychninization of the superior colliculus of cats. J. Neurophysiol. 9: 73-86, 1946.

Aschan, G., M. Bergstedt and J. Stahle: Nystagmography. Recording of nystagmus in clinical neuro-otological examinations. Acta Oto-Laryngol. Suppl. 129: 1-103, 1956.

Bailey, P., G. von Bonin, H. W. Garol and W. S. McCulloch: Functional organization of temporal lobe of monkey (Macaca mulatta) and chimpanzee (Pan satyrus). J. Neurophysiol. 6: 121-128, 1943.

Barnard, J. W.: The hypoglossal complex of vertebrates. J. Comp. Neur. 72: 489-524, 1940.

Barnes, W. T., H. W. Magoun and S. W. Ranson: The ascending auditory pathway in the brain stem of the monkey. J. Comp. Neur. 79: 129-152, 1943.

Berry, C. M., W. D. Hagamen and J. C. Hinsey: Distribution of potentials following stimulation of olfactory bulb in cat. J. Neurophysiol. 15: 139-148, 1952.

Björk, A. and E. Kugelberg: Motor unit activity in the human extraocular muscles. EEG and Clin. Neurophysiol. 5: 271-278, 1953a.

—— The electrical activity of the muscles of the eye and eyelids in various positions and during movement. EEG and Clin. Neurophysiol. 5: 595-602, 1953b.

Björkman, A. und G. Wohlfart: Faseranalyse der Nn. oculomotorius, trochlearis und abducens des Menschen und des N. abducens verschiedener Tiere. Z. mikr. anat. Forsch. 39: 631-647, 1936.

Boyd, J. D.: Observations on the human carotid sinus and its nerve supply. Anat. Anz. *84:* 386-399, 1937.

Brocklehurst, R. J. and F. H. Edgeworth: The fibre components of the laryngeal nerves of Macaca mulatta. J. Anat. *74:* 386-389, 1940.

Brodal, A.: Lammelse av m. rectus oculi externus som eneste utfallssymptom ved poliomyelitt. Nord. Med. *28:* 2332-2334, 1945.

—— Central course of afferent fibers for pain in facial, glossopharyngeal and vagus nerves. Arch. Neurol. Psychiat. *57:*292-306, 1947a.

—— The hippocampus and the sense of smell. Brain *70:* 179-222, 1947b.

—— The pyramidal tract in the light of recent anatomical research. Irish J. Med. Sci. pp. 289-302, 1953.

Brodal, A. and B. Høivik: Site and mode of termination of primary vestibulocerebellar fibres in the cat. An experimental study with silver impregnation methods. Arch. Ital. de Biol. *102:* 1-21, 1964.

Brodal, A. and O. Pompeiano: The vestibular nuclei in the cat. J. Anat. *91:* 438-454, 1957a.

—— The origin of ascending fibres of the medial longitudinal fasciculus from the vestibular nuclei. An experimental study in the cat. Acta Morphol. Neerlando-Scand. *1:* 306-328, 1957b.

Brodal, A. and A. Torvik: Über den Ursprung der sekundären vestibulocerebellaren Fasern bei der Katze. Arch. f. Psychiat. u. Z. Neur. *195:* 550-567, 1957.

Brodal, A., Th. Szabo and A. Torvik: Corticofugal fibers to sensory trigeminal nuclei and nucleus of solitary tract. An experimental study in the cat. J. Comp. Neur. *106:* 527-556, 1956.

Bruesch, S. R.: The distribution of myelinated afferent fibers in the branches of the cat's facial nerve. J. Comp. Neur. *81:* 169-191, 1944.

Bruesch, S. R. and L. B. Arey: The number of myelinated and unmyelinated fibers in the optic nerve of vertebrates. J. Comp. Neur. *77:* 631-665, 1942.

Buchanan, A. R.: The course of the secondary vestibular fibers in the cat. J. Comp. Neur. *67:* 183-204, 1937.

Buskirk, C. van: The seventh nerve complex. J. Comp. Neur. *82:* 303-333, 1945.

Börnstein, W. S.: Cortical representation of taste in man and monkey. II. The localization of the cortical taste area in man and a method of measuring impairment of taste in man. Yale J. Biol. Med. *13:* 133-156, 1940.

Carpenter, M. B. and R. R. McMasters: Disturbances of conjugate horizontal eye movements in the monkey. II. Physiological effects and anatomical degeneration resulting from lesions in the medial longitudinal fasciculus. Arch. Neurol. *8:* 347-368, 1963.

Clark, W. E. Le Gros and M. Meyer: The terminal connexions of the olfactory tract in the rabbit. Brain 70: 304-328, 1947.

Clark, W. E. Le Gros and G. G. Penman: The projection of the retina in the lateral geniculate body. Proc. Roy. Soc. Lond. Ser. B. 114: 291-313, 1934.

Cooper, S.: Muscle spindles in the intrinsic muscles of the human tongue. J. Physiol. 122: 193-202, 1953.

Cooper, S. and P. M. Daniel: Muscle spindles in human extrinsic eye muscles. Brain 72: 1-24, 1949.

Cooper, S., P. M. Daniel and D. Whitteridge: Afferent impulses in the oculomotor nerve from the extrinsic eye muscles. J. Physiol. 113: 463-474, 1951.

—— Nerve impulses in the brainstem of the goat. Short latency responses obtained by stretching the extrinsic eye muscles and the jaw muscles. J. Physiol. 120: 471-490, 1953a.

—— Nerve impulses in the brainstem of the goat. Responses with long latencies obtained by stretching the extrinsic eye muscles. J. Physiol. 120: 491-513, 1953b.

—— Nerve impulses in the brainstem and cortex of the goat. Spontaneous discharges and responses to visual and other afferent stimuli. J. Physiol. 120: 514-527, 1953c.

Corbin, K. B.: Observations on the peripheral distribution of fibers arising in the mesencephalic nucleus of the fifth cranial nerve. J. Comp. Neur. 73: 153-177, 1940.

Corbin, K. B. and F. Harrison: Function of mesencephalic root of the fifth cranial nerve. J. Neurophysiol. 3: 423-435, 1940.

Crosby, E. C.: Relations of brain centers to normal and abnormal eye movements in the horizontal plane. J. Comp. Neur. 99: 437-479, 1953.

Crosby, E. C. and J. W. Henderson: The mammalian midbrain and isthmus regions. II. Fiber connections of the superior colliculus. B. Pathways concerned in automatic eye movements. J. Comp. Neur. 88: 53-91, 1948.

Desmedt, J. E.: Neurophysiological mechanisms controlling acoustic input. Pp. 152-164 in Neural Mechanisms of the Auditory and Vestibular Systems. Ed. by Grant L. Rasmussen and William F. Windle, Charles C. Thomas, Springfield, Ill., 1960.

Dow, R. S.: The fiber connections of the posterior parts of the cerebellum in the cat and rat. J. Comp. Neur. 63: 527-548, 1936.

DuBois, F. S. and J. O. Foley: Experimental studies on the vagus and spinal accessory nerves in the cat. Anat. Rec. 64: 285-307, 1936.

—— Quantitative studies of the vagus nerve in the cat. II. The ratio of jugular to nodose fibers. J. Comp. Neur. 67: 69-87, 1937.

Elsberg, C. A. and I. Levy: The sense of smell. I. A new and simple method of quantitative olfactometry. Bull. Neur. Inst. New York. *4:* 5-19, 1935.

Falconer, M. A.: Intramedullary trigeminal tractotomy and its place in the treatment of facial pain. J. Neurol. Neurosurg. Psychiat. *12:* 297-311, 1949.

Feinstein, B., B. Lindegård, E. Nyman and G. Wohlfart: Morphologic studies of motor units in normal human muscles. Acta Anat. *23:* 127-142, 1954.

Fisher, C. M. and R. D. Adams: Diphtheritic polyneuritis—A pathological study. J. Neuropathol. Exp. Neurol. *15:* 243-268, 1956.

Foley, J. O. and F. DuBois: Quantitative studies of the vagus nerve in the cat. I. The ratio of sensory to motor fibers. J. Comp. Neur. *67:* 49-67, 1937.

—— An experimental study of the facial nerve. J. Comp. Neur. *79:* 79-105, 1943.

Gacek, R. R.: Efferent component of the vestibular nerve. Pp. 276-284 in Neural Mechanisms of the Auditory and Vestibular Systems. Ed. by Grant L. Rasmussen and William F. Windle, Charles C. Thomas, Springfield, Ill., 1960.

Gerebtzoff, M. A.: Les voies centrales de la sensibilité et du goût et leurs terminaisons thalamiques. La Cellule *48:*91-146, 1939.

Gernandt, B. E.: Vestibular mechanisms. Pp. 549-564 in Handbook of Physiology. Section I: Neurophysiology, vol. I. American Physiological Society, Washington, D.C. 1959.

Getz, B. and T. Sirnes: The localization within the dorsal motor vagal nucleus. An experimental investigation. J. Comp. Neur. *90:* 95-110, 1949.

Glees, P. and W. E. Le Gros Clark: The termination of optic fibres in the lateral geniculate body of the monkey. J. Anat. *75:* 295-308, 1941.

Hagbarth, K.-E. and D. I. B. Kerr: Central influences on spinal afferent conduction. J. Neurophysiol. *17:* 295-307, 1954.

Harrison, F. and K. B. Corbin: Oscillographic studies on the spinal tract of the fifth cranial nerve. J. Neurophysiol. *5:* 465-482, 1942.

Hernández-Peón, R. and K.-E. Habgarth: Interaction between afferent and cortically induced reticular responses. J. Neurophysiol. *18:* 44-55, 1955.

Herrick, C. J.: The cranial nerves. A review of fifty years. Denison Univ. Bull. J. Sci. Lab. *38:* 41-51, 1943.

Holmes, G.: The cerebral integration of ocular movements. Brit. Med. J. 1938, II: 107-112.

Humphrey, T. A.: The development of the olfactory and accessory olfactory formation in human embryos and fetuses. J. Comp. Neur. *73:* 431-468, 1940.

Ingram, W. R. and E. A. Dawkins: The intramedullary course of afferent fibers of the vagus nerve in the cat. J. Comp. Neur. *82:* 157-168, 1945.

Kaada, B. R., J. Jansen Jr. and P. Andersen: Stimulation of the hippocampus and medial cortical areas in unanesthetized cats. Neurology *3:* 844-857, 1953.

Kiloh, L. G. and S. Nevin: Progressive dystrophy of the external ocular muscles (Ocular myopathy). Brain *74:* 115-143, 1951.

Kristensen, H. K. and K. Zilstorff-Pedersen: Quantitative studies on the function of smell. Acta Oto-Laryngol. *43:* 537-544, 1953.

Kristiansen, K.: Et pedunkulært kalott-syndrom. Nord. Med. *8:* 22-41, 1940.

Kuypers, H. G. J. M.: Corticobulbar connexions to the pons and lower brain-stem in man. An anatomical study. Brain *81:* 364-388, 1958.

Lassek, A. M.: The human pyramidal tract. II. A numerical investigation of the Betz cells of the motor area. Arch. Neurol. Psychiat. *44:* 718-724, 1940.

—— The pyramidal tract. The effect of pre- and postcentral cortical lesions on the fiber components of the pyramids in monkey. J. Nerv. Ment. Dis. *95:* 721-729, 1942.

Lewy, F. H. and H. Kobrak: The neural projection of the cochlear spirals on the primary acoustic centers. Arch. Neurol. Psychiat. *35:* 839-852, 1936.

Löwenstein, O. and A. Sand: The mechanism of the semicircular canal. A study of the responses of single-fibre preparations to angular accelerations and to rotation at constant speed. Proc. Roy. Soc. Lond. Ser. B *129:* 256-275, 1940.

Magoun, H. W.: The ascending reticular system and wakefulness. Pp. 1-15 in Brain Mechanisms and Consciousness. Ed. by J. F. Delafresnaye. Blackwell, Oxford, 1954.

Magoun, H. W. and S. W. Ranson: The afferent path of the light reflex. A review of the literature. Arch. Ophthal. *13:* 862-874, 1935.

Meyer, M. and A. C. Allison: An experimental investigation of the connexions of the olfactory tracts in monkey. J. Neurol. Neurosurg. Psychiat. *12:* 274-286, 1949.

Monrad-Krohn, G. H.: On the dissociation of voluntary and emotional innervation in facial paresis of central origin. Brain *47:* 22-37, 1924.

Moore, R. Y. and J. M. Goldberg: Ascending projections of the inferior colliculus in the cat. J. Comp. Neur. *121:* 109-135, 1963.

Moruzzi, G. and H. W. Magoun: Brain stem reticular formation and activation of the EEG. EEG Clin. Neurophysiol. *1:* 455-473, 1949.

Müller, R. and G. Wohlfart: Om tumörer i corpus pineale (Pinea tumors). Nord. Med. *33:* 15-21, 1947.

Nicolaissen, B. and A. Brodal: Chronic progressive external ophthalmoplegia. Report of a case with histopathologic examination of external eye muscle and skeletal muscle. A.M.A. Arch. Ophthalm. *61:* 203-211, 1959.

Nyberg-Hansen, R.: Origin and termination of fibres from the vestibular nuclei descending in the medial longitudinal fasciculus. An experimental study with silver impregnation methods in the cat. J. Comp. Neur. *122:* 355-367, 1964.

Nyberg-Hansen, R. and T. A. Mascitti: Sites and mode of termination of fibers of the vestibulo-spinal tract in the cat. An experimental study with silver impregnation methods. J. Comp. Neur. *122:* 369-387, 1964.

Ogura, J. H. and R. L. Lam: Anatomical and physiological correlations on stimulating the human superior laryngeal nerve. Laryngoscope *63:* 947-959, 1953.

Olivecrona, H.: Tractotomy for relief of trigeminal neuralgia. Arch. Neurol. Psychiat. *47:* 544-564, 1942.

Olszewski, J.: On the anatomical and functional organization of the spinal trigeminal nucleus. J. Comp. Neur. *92:* 401-413, 1950.

Patton, H. D., T. C. Ruch and A. E. Walker: Experimental hypogeusia from Horsley-Clarke lesions of the thalamus in macaca mulatta. J. Neurophysiol. *7:* 171-184. 1944.

Pearson, A. A.: The spinal accessory nerve in human embryos. J. Comp. Neur. *68:* 243-266, 1938.

—— The development of the nervus terminalis in man. J. Comp. Neur. *75:* 39-66, 1941.

—— Observations on the roots of the facial nerve in human fetuses. Anat. Rec. *91:* 294-295, 1945.

—— The development and connections of the mesencephalic root of the trigeminal nerve in man. J. Comp. Neur. *90:* 1-46, 1949a.

—— Further observations on the mesencephalic root of the trigeminal nerve. J. Comp. Neur. *91:* 147-194, 1949b.

Pfaffmann, C.: Afferent impulses from the teeth due to pressure and noxious stimulation. J. Physiol. *97:* 207-219, 1939.

Pompeiano, A. and A. Brodal: The origin of vestibulospinal fibres in the cat. An experimental-anatomical study, with comments on the descending medial longitudinal fasciculus. Arch. Ital. de Biol. *95:* 166-195, 1957a.

—— Spinovestibular fibers in the cat. An experimental study. J. Comp. Neur. *108:* 353-381, 1957b.

Pompeiano, O. and F. Walberg: Descending connections to the vestibular nuclei. An experimental study in the cat. J. Comp. Neur. *108:* 465-502, 1957.

Rasmussen, A. T. and W. T. Peyton: Origin of the ventral external arcuate fibers and their continuity with the striae medullares of the fourth ventricle of man. J. Comp. Neur. *84:* 325-337, 1946

Rasmussen, G. L.: The olivary peduncle and other fiber projections of the superior olivary complex. J. Comp. Neur. *84:* 141-220, 1946.

—— Further observations of the efferent cochlear bundle. J. Comp. Neur. *99:* 61-74, 1953.

Rose, J. E., R. Galambos and J. R. Hughes: Microelectrode studies of the cochlear nuclei of the cat. Bull Johns Hopkins Hosp. *104:* 211-251, 1959.

Rossi, G. F. and A. Zanchetti: The brain stem reticular formation. Anatomy and physiology. Arch. Ital. de Biol. *95:* 199-435, 1957.

Russell, G. V.: The dorsal trigemino-thalamic tract in the cat reconsidered as a lateral reticulo-thalamic system of connections. J. Comp. Neur. *101:* 237-264, 1954.

Schwartz, H. D., G. E. Roulhac, R. L. Lam and J. O'Leary: Organization of the fasciculus solitarius in man. J. Comp. Neur. *94:* 221-237, 1951.

Schwarz, G. A. and C.-N. Liu: Chronic progressive external ophthalmoplegia. A.M.A. Arch. Neurol. Psychiat. *71:* 31-53, 1954.

Schwarz, H. G. and G. Weddell: Observations on the pathways transmitting the sensation of taste. Brain *61:* 99-115, 1938.

Shute, C. C. D.: The anatomy of the eighth cranial nerve in man. Proc. Roy. Soc. Med. *44:* 1013-1018, 1951.

Smyth, G. E.: The systematization and central connections of the spinal tract and nucleus of the trigeminal nerve. A clinical and pathological study. Brain *62:* 41-87, 1939.

Stotler, W. A.: An experimental study of the cells and connections of the superior olivary complex of the cat. J. Comp. Neur. *98:* 401-432, 1953.

Sunderland, S.: Neurovascular relations and anomalies at the base of the brain. J. Neurol. Neurosurg. Psychiat. *11:* 243-257, 1948.

Sunderland, S. and K. C. Bradley: Disturbances of oculomotor function accompanying extradural haemorrhage. J. Neurol. Neurosurg. Psychiat. *16:* 35-46, 1953.

Sunderland, S. and D. F. Cossar: The structure of the facial nerve. Anat. Rec. *116:* 147-165, 1953.

Sunderland, S. and E. S. R. Hughes: The pupillo-constrictor pathway and the nerves to the ocular muscles in man. Brain *69:* 301-309, 1946.

Sunderland, S. and W. E. Swaney: The intraneural topography of the recurrent laryngeal nerve in man. Anat. Rec. *114:* 411-426, 1952.

Szentágothai, J.: Die innere Gliederung des Oculomotoriuskernes. Arch. f. Psychiat. *115:* 127-135, 1942a.

—— Die zentrale Leitungsbahn des Lichtreflexes der Pupillen. Arch. f. Psychiat. *115:* 136-156, 1942b.

—— Die Lokalisation der Kehlkopfmuskulatur in den Vaguskernen. Z. Anat. u. Entw.gesch. *112:* 704-710, 1943a.

—— Die zentrale Innervation der Augenbewegungen. Arch f. Psychiat. *116:* 721-760, 1943b.

—— Anatomical considerations of monosynaptic reflex arcs. J. Neurophysiol. *11:* 445-454, 1948a.

—— The representation of facial and scalp muscles in the facial nucleus. J. Comp. Neur. *88:* 207-220, 1948b.

—— Functional representation in the motor trigeminal nucleus. J. Comp. Neur. *90:* 111-120, 1949.

Szentágothai, J. and K. Rajkovits: Der Hirnnervenanteil der Pyramidenbahn und der prämotorische Apparat motorischer Hirnnervenkerne. Arch. Psychiat. u. Ztschr. ges. Neur. *197:* 335-354, 1958.

Tarkhan, A. A.: The innervation of the extrinsic ocular muscles. J. Anat. *68:* 293-313, 1934.

Tarkhan, A. A. and S. A. El-Malek: On the presence of sensory nerve cells on the hypoglossal nerve. J. Comp. Neur. *93:* 219-228, 1950.

Taverner, D.: Bell's palsy. A clinical and electromyographic study. Brain *78:* 209-228, 1955.

Torvik, A.: Afferent connections to the sensory trigeminal nuclei, the nucleus of the solitary tract and adjacent structures. J. Comp. Neur. *106:* 51-141, 1956.

—— Die Lokalisation des 'Speichelzentrums' bei der Katze. Z. mikr.-anat. Forsch. *63:* 317-326, 1957a.

—— The ascending fibers from the main trigeminal sensory nucleus. An experimental study in the cat. Am. J. Anat. *100:* 1-16, 1957b.

Torvik, A. and A. Brodal: The cerebellar projection of the perihypoglossal nuclei (nucleus intercalatus, nucleus praepositus hypoglossi and nucleus of Roller) in the cat. J. Neuropath. Exp. Neur. *13:* 515-527, 1954.

Tunturi, A. R.: Physiological determination of the arrangement of the afferent connections to the middle ectosylvian auditory area in the dog. Am. J. Physiol. *162:* 489-502, 1950.

Walberg, F.: Corticofugal fibres to the nuclei of the dorsal columns. An experimental study in the cat. Brain *80:* 273-287, 1957a.

—— Do the motor nuclei of the cranial nerves receive corticofugal fibres? An experimental study in the cat. Brain *80:* 597-605, 1957b.

Walberg, F., D. Bowsher and A. Brodal: The termination of primary vestibular fibres in the vestibular nuclei in the cat. An experimental study with silver methods. J. Comp. Neur. *110:* 391-419, 1958.

Walberg, F. and A. Brodal: Pyramidal tract fibres from temporal and occipital lobes. An experimental study in the cat. Brain *76:* 491-508, 1953.

Walker, A. E.: The origin, course and terminations of the secondary pathways of the trigeminal nerve in primates. J. Comp. Neur. *71:* 59-89, 1939.

Walker, A. E. and J. F. Fulton: The thalamus of the chimpanzee. III. Metathalamus. Normal structure and cortical connections. Brain *61:* 250-268, 1938.

Warwick, R.: Representation of the extra-ocular muscles in the oculomotor nuclei of the monkey. J. Comp. Neur. *98:* 449-503, 1953.

—— The ocular parasympathetic nerve supply and its mesencephalic sources. J. Anat. *88:* 71-93, 1954.

Weddell, G., B. Feinstein and R. E. Pattle: The electrical activity of voluntary muscle in man under normal and pathological conditions. Brain *67:* 178-257, 1944.

Subject Index

When a subject is treated on more than one page ff after the figure indicates the place where it is most completely described. f indicates reference to a footnote.